NEONATAL IMAGING

NEONATAL IMAGING

FIRST EDITION

Developmental Editor
Robin L. Bissinger, PhD, APRN, NNP-BC, FAAN
Executive Director
The National Certification Corporation (NCC)
Chicago, Illinois

Author and Editor
Meryle J. Eklund, MD
Assistant Professor of Radiology and Pediatrics
Department of Radiology and Radiological Science
Medical University of South Carolina
Charleston, South Carolina

Authors
Jeanne G. Hill, MD
Professor of Radiology and Pediatrics
Department of Radiology and Radiological Science
Medical University of South Carolina
Charleston, South Carolina

Caroline C. Swift, MD
Radiology Resident
Department of Radiology and Radiological Science
Medical University of South Carolina
Charleston, South Carolina

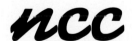

THE NATIONAL CERTIFICATION CORPORATION
CHICAGO

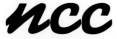
The National Certification Corporation
676 N. Michigan Ave., Ste. 3600
Chicago, Illinois 60611

Neonatal Imaging ISBN: 978-0-9890198-2-8
© 2018 by National Certification Corporation.

All Rights Reserved. No part of this publication may be reproduced or transmitted by any means, electronic or mechanical, including photocopying, recording, or otherwise, without written permission from the publisher. For information, write National Certification Corporation, 676 N. Michigan Ave., Suite 3600, Chicago, Illinois 60611.

This book and the individual contributions contained in it are protected by copyright by the Publisher (except as noted herein).

Notices

While all reasonable effort has been made to assure both accuracy and timeliness of the information in this publication, new evidence and research continually impact practice. The authors, editors, and publishers do not take responsibility for the accuracy or completeness of any of the information contained herein and it is expected that providers utilize the most current information, policies, and guidelines at their practice sites for the care of patients.

This book and the authors, editors, and publishers recognize that this publication contains information on health care that is intended for use as assistance only to the professional practitioner. The actual use of, and interpretation of, this information is solely the responsibility of the practitioner.

Although case histories are drawn from actual cases, every effort has been made to disguise the identities of the individuals involved.

Any reference to any procedure, device, drug, or drug dosage (unless otherwise indicated in the text) is based on the generally accepted standards in effect at the time of publication and, if applicable, reflects the then current FDA-approved usages for drugs and devices. Since such standards and usages are subject to change and interpretation based on research and new information, it is the responsibility of any practitioner to check the applicable current standards and FDA usage recommendations prior to use in practice.

The editors, authors, and publishers disclaim any responsibility for any adverse effects resulting from the suggested procedures, from any undetected errors, or from the reader's misunderstanding of the text.

Library of Congress Cataloging-in-Publication Data
Personal name: Eklund, Meryle J.
Main title: Neonatal Imaging / Meryle J. Eklund, MD, Jeanne G. Hill, MD, Caroline C. Swift, MD; [edited by] Robin L. Bissinger, PhD, APRN, NNP-BC, FAAN, Meryle J. Eklund, MD.
Edition: 1st edition.
Published/Produced: Chicago, IL: National Certification Corporation, 2018. | includes index.
Identifiers: LCCN 2017962756 (print) | ISBN: 9780989019828 (pbk. : alk. paper)
Subjects: Pediatrics –Newborn infants | Neonatology –Diseases and abnormalities –Examination | Diagnosis – Special diagnostic methods, A-Z –Radiography | Diagnosis –Special diagnostic methods, A-Z –Diagnostic imaging | Neonatology – methods | Handbooks
Classification:
LC record available at https://lccn.loc.gov/2017962756

Developmental Editor: Robin L. Bissinger, PhD, APRN, NNP-BC, FAAN
Editor: Meryle J. Eklund, MD
Project & Publishing Services Manager: Cyndi Scovel
Medical Editor: Jennifer Moore
Cover Design: Handel Design
Page Design: Mary T. Burke
Illustrations: Lobsang Studio

Printed in the United States of America.
10 9 8 7 6 5 4 3 2 1

Foreword

Neonatal health care providers are faced with the challenge of keeping up with the "state of the science." We are expected to have mastered a foundation of knowledge and to build on it continually. In today's age of data and technology, advances in neonatal imaging will expand our understanding of neonatal disease and alter how we diagnose and treat our patients. *Neonatal Imaging* provides the foundation for neonatal health care providers to understand the techniques, artifacts and positioning; to relate detailed pathology and the interpretation of neonatal radiologic and sonographic images; and to differentiate between normal and abnormal findings vs. artifact. It creates a framework for neonatal imaging, providing both basic and challenging issues when reading and interpreting x-rays and ultrasounds.

Although the term "neonatology" was not introduced until 1960, many of the principles and practices in use today have roots that go back much further. The 19th century brought about the discovery of many new technologies, including the development of both incubators and x-rays. Both of these discoveries would dramatically alter the care provided to critically ill infants. The initial work with premature and critically ill infants started with nurse midwives and obstetricians in France and evolved with "incubator sideshows" at expositions and World's Fairs as early as 1898. These shows were designed initially to demonstrate the new technology of the incubator, and in time, this new technology would become a standard of care that would save the lives of premature infants.

The use of incubators and temperature regulation, founded in Europe as early as 1835, would be realized as lifesaving support by the 1950s. Around 1895, x-rays would also be discovered, becoming a routine part of medical practice by 1896. However, it would not be until 1910, with the publication of a book about radiology in children, that radiology as a subspecialty would begin to evolve along with progress in pediatric radiology. In addition, in 1923, a physician named J.W. Ballantyne was the first to discuss the need for "specialization in neonatal medicine," pointing out that trained experts were essential to the care of these unique patients. This would begin a journey in pediatric subspecialties with a focus on neonatal medicine.

It wasn't until 1945, when a revolutionary text of pediatric x-ray diagnosis was published, that pediatric radiology would begin to progress and revolutionize the field over the next 50 years. The first fellowship in pediatric radiology was granted in 1949 and led to ongoing improvements in imaging, especially of the chest and abdomen, that allowed radiographic examination of newborns to become feasible. The first neonatal intensive care unit was developed in the 1960s, along with lifesaving technologies such as laboratory evaluation, fluid and electrolyte management, and respiratory support, that were specific to this very vulnerable population. Ultrasound imaging, developed in 1957, was first used in children in 1974. Both CT and MRI modalities were invented in the 1970s and were being used in pediatrics by 1975. Pediatric radiology and the care of neonates continues to explode and expand and the technology we use today will advance uniquely in years to come.

As a nurse practitioner and researcher, the care of premature and critically ill neonates has been my passion for my entire career. A strong foundational knowledge of normal physiology and available technologies that impact care is critical to understand the difficulties these vulnerable infants face, to question practice, and to develop and initiate treatments that meet their needs. As an educator, I have found that students must be able to discuss both the normal and abnormal findings when assessing a critically ill neonate. Neonatal imaging requires an understanding of what normal findings look like and how normal and abnormal findings can be related to different illnesses. The ability to observe subtle changes in a normal image, noting artifacts, penetration, positioning and line issues; can better focus the provider on the abnormality of the image that leads to the correct conclusion.

The authors of this book are faculty at a large, regional, referral medical center. They have years of experience in neonatal and pediatric imaging. In addition, they are colleagues, national leaders, and friends. The dedication of these authors in volunteering their time and resources to provide readers with a detailed understanding of imaging, specific to the neonate, is evident in each chapter. *Neonatal Imaging* discusses the basic principles of common neonatal imaging studies, the pathophysiology of pertinent diseases, and the challenges in reading and evaluating findings. It was written as a learning tool for students and new providers, and as a resource for skilled clinicians.

Over the centuries, new developments and techniques have changed the face of pediatric and neonatal health care. From smaller hand-held devices to non-invasive technologies, imaging studies will become easier and more accurate. Scanned images of the soft and hard tissues of the body will offer such detail that they could eliminate the need for exploratory surgeries and other invasive procedures. Imaging in the future may be able to detect disease earlier.

Health care professionals and medical and nursing students are challenged to acquire and maintain expertise in all areas of their practice. Information expands at a rapid pace and challenges the best of us. In 2010, it was estimated that knowledge doubles every 3.5 years and is estimated to double every 73 days by 2020. Knowledge expands faster than our ability to assimilate and apply it effectively. What is key is an expectation that providers have a foundational knowledge that they have mastered and that they build on this continually. This text is dedicated to increasing knowledge of neonatal imaging and is designed for neonatal health care providers along a continuum from new learner to expert clinician.

Robin L. Bissinger, PhD, APRN, NNP-BC, FAAN
Executive Director
The National Certification Corporation (NCC)
Chicago, Illinois

Preface

Neonates may be affected by a wide variety of conditions, ranging from prematurity to congenital anomalies to acquired illnesses. Each of these vulnerable infants require a heightened level of evaluation and care, in which imaging plays a vital role. Multiple imaging examinations are often necessary to aid in diagnosis and help guide clinical management.

The purpose of this book is to provide a better understanding of the basics of imaging and the language of radiology to aid clinicians in the evaluation of neonates. *Neonatal Imaging* places particular emphasis on radiography and sonography, two of the principle imaging modalities used in everyday neonatal care. A sound appreciation of why images look the way they do will help readers learn how to recognize abnormalities independently and gain a deeper understanding of the diagnostic workups of sick infants.

Neonatal Imaging presents many excellent examples of imaging studies you can expect to see in a neonatal intensive care unit or a newborn nursery. Although we discuss basic imaging principles, this book is not an exhaustive review of the subject and does not cover many important topics that are beyond its scope. Therefore, be sure to consult your institution's radiologists to confirm any findings you discover, if you have questions regarding the appropriate utilization of imaging, and in complex cases.

Meryle J. Eklund, MD
Jeanne G. Hill, MD
Caroline C. Swift, MD

Acknowledgements

We would like to thank our peer reviewers for their contributions to the development of *Neonatal Imaging*.

Margaret Conway-Orgel, DNP, NNP-BC
Neonatal Nurse Practitioner
Medical University of South Carolina
Charleston, South Carolina

Rebecca J. McPherson, MD, FAAP
Neonatal-Perinatal Medicine, Board Certified
Neonatologist
KIDZ Medical Services at Martin Memorial Health System
Stuart, Florida

Stephen F. Simoneaux, MD
Associate Professor, Department of Radiology and Imaging Sciences
Emory University
Atlanta, Georgia
Chief of Radiology
Children's Healthcare of Atlanta
Atlanta, Georgia

Ted S. Wen, MD, FACR
Pediatric Radiologist
Managing Partner
Texas Radiology Associates, LLP
Dallas, Texas

Images courtesy of the Department of Radiology and Radiological Sciences at the Medical University of South Carolina.

Contents

Introduction: Terms And Techniques 1

1. **The Neonatal Chest**
   Technique 7
   Positioning 10
   Normal Chest Radiograph 14
   Lung Volumes 18
   Lines and Tubes 21
   The Periphery 35
   Pathology 39

2. **The Neonatal Abdomen**
   Technique 87
   Positioning 88
   Normal Abdominal Radiograph 90
   Lines and Tubes 92
   The Periphery: Bones and Soft Tissues 113
   Pathology 119

3. **The Neonatal Head**
   Technique 165
   Normal Head Ultrasound 167
   Pathology 171

4. **The Neonatal Urinary Tract**
   Technique 201
   Normal Kidney Ultrasound 202
   Pathology 204

5. **Artifacts**
   Skin Folds 223
   Mach Effect 225
   Monitoring Leads and Devices 227
   Clothing and Diapers 229
   Comfort Items 231
   Other External Artifacts 232

6. **Case Challenges** 235

Appendix: Glossary Of Acronyms 277
Suggested Resources 279
Index 281

Introduction Terms and Techniques

A solid understanding of the terms and techniques used in radiology is necessary when interpreting neonatal imaging. This Introduction provides a review of some of the more important common nomenclature as discussed in this book.

IONIZING RADIATION

When ordering radiologic examinations – especially for neonates – it is of utmost importance to take into account whether the procedure requires the use of **ionizing radiation**, as well as the relative radiation exposure to the patient. Pediatric patients are up to 10 times more susceptible to radiation-induced cellular damage than adults and have a longer projected lifetime in which complications can manifest. Due to its association with an increased risk of malignancy and other harmful effects, exposure to ionizing radiation should be limited.

Plain radiographs and basic fluoroscopic studies use modern low-dose techniques associated with very low radiation exposure. Lengthy fluoroscopic procedures, such as cardiac catheterization and certain nuclear medicine studies, can expose the patient to tens to hundreds of times the dose of a single radiograph. Computed tomography (CT) also utilizes ionizing radiation, but the dose will depend on the body part that is scanned and the technique that is used. Since ultrasound and magnetic resonance imaging (MRI) do not use ionizing radiation, these forms do not carry the same risks.

The **ALARA (As Low As Reasonably Achievable) principle**, in which every reasonable effort to limit exposure to ionizing radiation is employed, is strongly endorsed by the pediatric medical imaging community. There are multiple ways to work toward this end in everyday practice:

- Never order a radiologic exam that will not alter management.
- Consider ultrasound or MRI modalities rather than those which utilize ionizing radiation.
- Use low-dose techniques when performing radiographic and fluoroscopic examinations.
- Image only the area of concern and avoid duplicate studies if the patient's clinical status has not changed.

While radiographic studies have great potential to facilitate management and improve patient outcomes, appropriate use of imaging techniques is essential to attain the safest environment for the infants in our care.

RADIOGRAPHIC IMAGING

An **x-ray** is electromagnetic wave of high energy and very short wavelength that is able to pass through many opaque and translucent materials. A **radiograph** is an image produced by x-rays that is used in medical examination. Therefore, when discussing imaging modalities, refer to a "chest radiograph," not a "chest x-ray."

Radiographs are interpreted based on assessing different densities:

> A **density** is an area of tissue on a radiograph that absorbs more x-rays instead of allowing them to pass through, creating a whiter area on the image. For example, bones are very dense tissue and will absorb x-rays. Therefore they appear lighter on the image.

> A **lucency** is an area of tissue that is less dense and allows x-rays to pass through easily, creating a darker area on a radiograph. For example, a healthy neonate's lungs are filled with air and less dense than surrounding tissue. Therefore, they appear darker, or more lucent, on the image.

Radiographs can be obtained in multiple projections to assess common problems:

Anteroposterior View

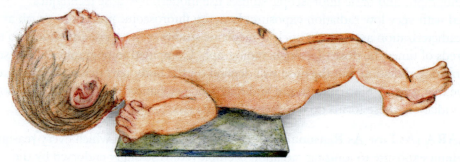

©2017 The National Certification Corporation

An **anteroposterior** radiograph is obtained with the patient lying on his or her back on the cassette and the x-ray tube positioned in front. This is the most common type of neonatal radiograph.

Posteroanterior View

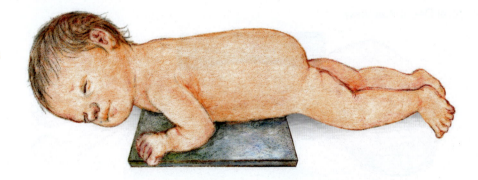

A **posteroanterior** radiograph is obtained with the patient lying on his or her stomach on the cassette and the x-ray tube positioned in back. This is less commonly used than anteroposterior views in neonates.

Cross-Table Lateral View

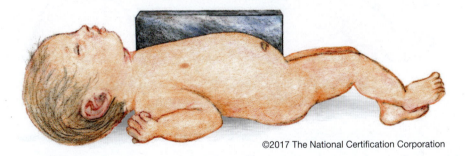

©2017 The National Certification Corporation

A **cross-table lateral** radiograph is obtained with the patient lying on his or her back. The image is typically acquired with the x-ray tube on the infant's right side and the cassette on the left side. This helps to localize findings seen on a frontal view of a neonate who cannot be repositioned or rotated. Cross-table lateral views may also be used to see where gas collects in patients with suspected pneumothorax or pneumoperitoneum.

Decubitus View

Right-Lateral Decubitus View

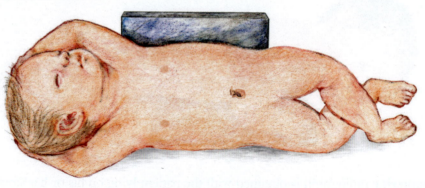

Left-Lateral Decubitus View

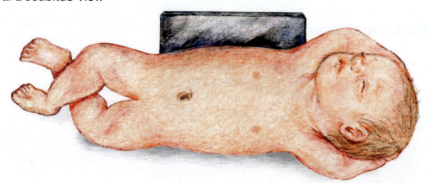

©2017 The National Certification Corporation

A **decubitus** radiograph is obtained with the patient lying on his or her right or left side and the cassette placed either anteriorly or posteriorly. These help to evaluate for the presence of free air in cases of pneumoperitoneum or pneumothorax, or for layering fluid in cases of pleural effusion.

ULTRASOUND IMAGING

Ultrasound is sound-wave energy that has a frequency higher than the range of human hearing. **Sonography** is the analysis of ultrasound using a machine that produces a graphical representation of its component frequencies.

Ultrasound examinations are interpreted by assessing the **echogenicity** of different tissues. Just as when interpreting radiographs, the ability of different tissues to transmit sound waves will produce different patterns on ultrasound.

> Substances that block transmission of sound waves, like bone, gas, or fat, will appear more **hyperechoic** (or brighter) than the surrounding tissue.

> Substances that easily transmit sound waves, like renal medulla or fluid, will be more **hypoechoic** (or darker) than the surrounding tissue.

Areas that lack echogenicity altogether, like a simple cyst or a simple fluid collection, will appear **anechoic**, or completely dark.

Tissue that has the same echogenicity as its surrounding tissue is described as **isoechoic**. For example, the caudate and the thalamus in a neonate normally have the same echogenicity and are therefore described as isoechoic to each other.

Doppler is a technique used in sonography to detect and measure blood flow within a mass or a vessel. Doppler can be used to assess velocity and flow characteristics.

COMPUTED TOMOGRAPHY (CT) IMAGING

CT is another imaging tool used to gather diagnostic information about patients. CT uses x-rays to obtain multiple radiographic images simultaneously and produce cross-sectional images of the body part being examined. CT images are particularly useful in evaluating large or complex anatomic abnormalities. They are obtained in the axial plane and reconstructed into the sagittal and coronal planes.

MAGNETIC RESONANCE IMAGING (MRI)

MRI is an advanced method that uses magnetic fields and radio waves to evaluate changes in the body's tissues. It can obtain both anatomic and physiologic information. MRI does not utilize ionizing radiation, which is a major benefit, but examinations are long and imaging is very sensitive to patient motion.

FLUOROSCOPIC IMAGING

Fluoroscopy is the use of x-rays to study moving structures. A continuous x-ray beam is passed through the pertinent body part, transmitting images to a monitor that allows evaluation of the organ and its surrounding movement in real time. Images are captured for more detailed evaluation at the workstation and for storage.

Contrast materials are used to increase the intrinsic visibility of structures that would be poorly seen by imaging alone. For example, oral contrast used in fluoroscopic imaging outlines the bowel lumen to demonstrate gastrointestinal anatomy that may not be visible on an x-ray image.

These fluoroscopic procedures are common for neonatal patients:

Upper gastrointestinal (UGI) exams are commonly performed to assess congenital malformations of the GI tract. An enteric contrast agent is used to evaluate the esophagus, stomach, and proximal small bowel. Multiple projections with the patient in different positions may be obtained to localize specific findings or to capitalize on the properties of gravity.

Voiding cystourethrograms (VCUGs) are commonly used to assess for functional and anatomic issues in the neonatal urinary system. A sterile catheter is used to allow water-soluble contrast to flow by gravity into the patient's bladder. During filling and distention of the bladder, the infant can be evaluated for anatomical abnormalities such as ureteroceles and posterior urethral valves, as well as functional or anatomical malformations leading to reflux.

SELECTION FACTORS

Certain strengths and weaknesses of the different imaging types are often taken into account when determining which type of procedure to be used. The table below summarizes the relative benefits and drawbacks of each modality in terms of radiation exposure, cost, need for sedation, time requirement, and real-time imaging capabilities.

COMPARISON TABLE OF IMAGING MODALITIES

Modality	Ionizing Radiation	Cost	Sedation	Time Requirement	Real-time Imaging
Radiography	+	$	-	+	-
Ultrasound	-	$$	-	++	+
CT	++	$$$	+/-	++	-
MRI	-	$$$$	+/-	++++	-
Fluoroscopy	+	$$	-	++	+

+ = present; - = absent

Chapter 1 The Neonatal Chest

TECHNIQUE

After confirming that the study corresponds to the correct patient, the first consideration when evaluating chest radiographs is image quality, or technique. Although obtaining adequate tissue penetration was more problematic before digital imaging display allowed the adjustment of image contrast and brightness at the workstation, it is still important.

Adequate Penetration

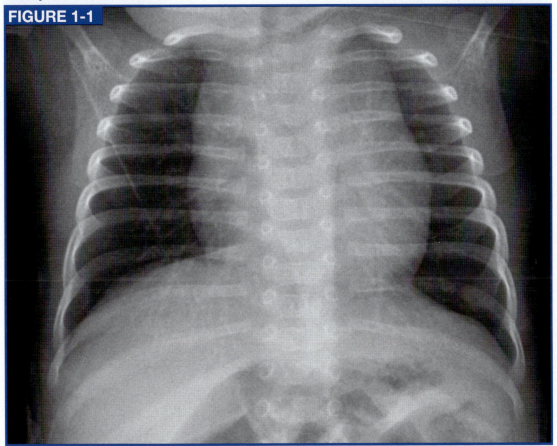

FIGURE 1-1

Adequate penetration allows visualization of the intervertebral disc spaces through the heart and of the pulmonary vasculature in the central third of the lungs.

Over-Penetration

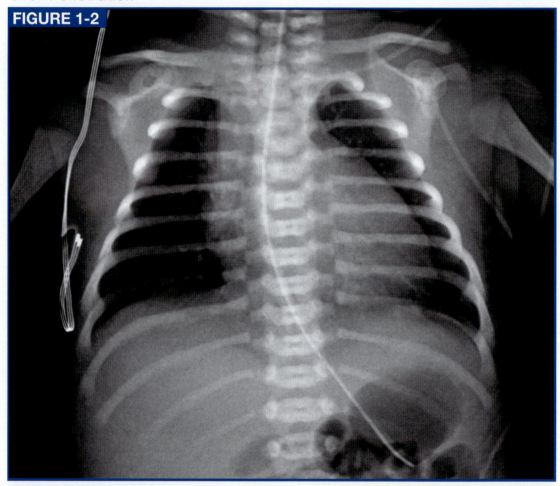

FIGURE 1-2

In an over-penetrated image, the lungs appear very dark and the pulmonary vasculature is difficult to see in the central third of the chest.

Under-Penetration

FIGURE 1-3

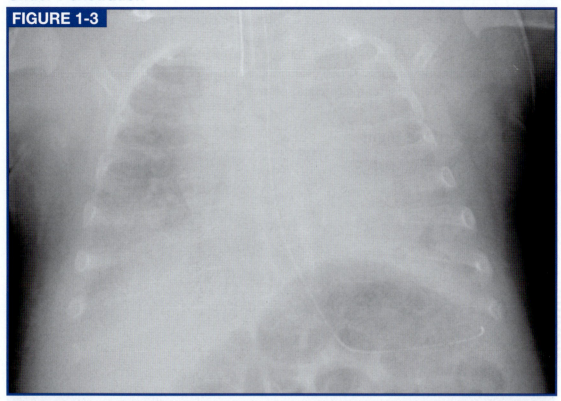

In an under-penetrated image, the spine is difficult to visualize through the heart. There is a generalized increased density of the lungs and soft tissues.

POSITIONING

The second consideration when evaluating a study is the patient's positioning. Slight rotation toward the right or left can significantly alter the projection of key structures and compromise the examination. Unfortunately, it is often difficult to correctly place and keep neonates in optimal position during imaging. When evaluating a study, try to determine whether rotation is present and how it could alter interpretation.

Rotation Toward the Right

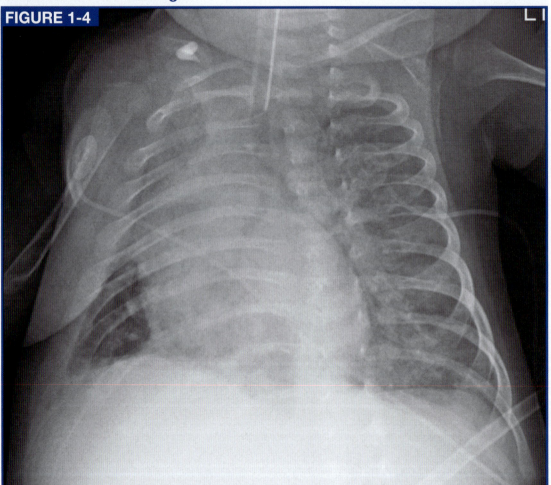

FIGURE 1-4

This patient is rotated significantly toward the right. Asymmetry of the clavicles and ribs is evident. The mediastinal structures project over the right chest. Note the elevation of the clavicle on the left and the longer appearance of the ribs on the right. It can be quite challenging to evaluate the lung parenchyma in patients who are rotated. In this image, the rotation makes the patient's heart and airway appear to be shifted to the right.

Rotation Toward the Left

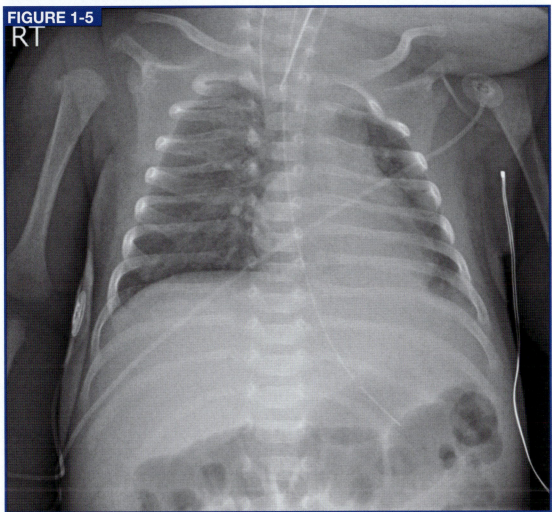

FIGURE 1-5

This patient is rotated toward the left. Again, the clavicles and ribs are asymmetric and the mediastinal structures project over the left chest. Note the elevated clavicle on the right side and the elongated appearance of the ribs on the left. In addition, the head is rotated toward the left, which makes the endotracheal tube tip appear higher. The tip will move slightly toward the carina when the head is facing forward.

Example of Displaced Sternal Ossification Centers Due to Rotation

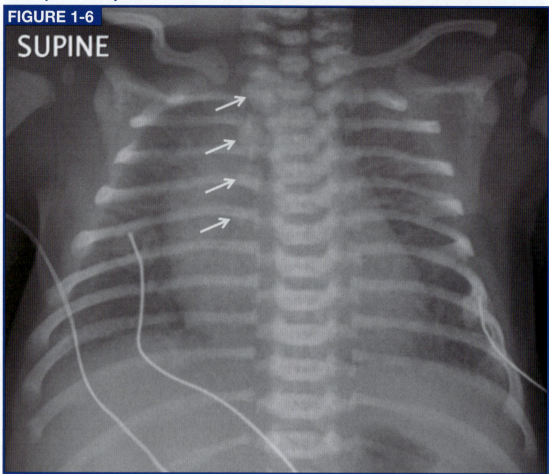

FIGURE 1-6

In this patient who is rotated toward the right, four well-defined, round, calcified structures project over the first through fourth right costovertebral junctions and medial ribs (arrows). They represent the sternal ossification centers, deviated to the right due to rotation, which can sometimes be mistaken for healing rib fractures.

The trajectory of the x-ray beam used to acquire an image is also important. Ideally, the center of the beam should be directed at the center of the chest. Mild deviation of the beam from the center of the target structure could result in significant distortion of the image.

Example of X-Ray Beam Trajectory Distortion

FIGURE 1-7

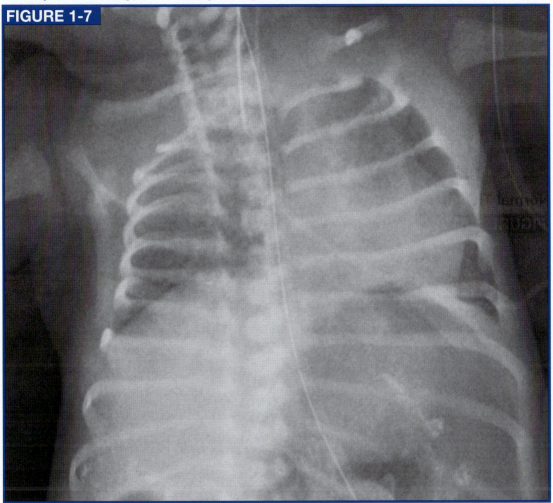

This patient is significantly rotated toward the left. In addition, the x-ray beam is focused on the left paramedian upper abdomen rather than the center of the chest and is directed superiorly toward the head, making the ribs and mediastinum appear stretched and shifted upward. In radiology, this is referred to as a lordotic projection. When the x-ray beam is pointed toward the head instead of perpendicular to the chest, the heart apex may also appear tilted upward. Note that the clavicles are elevated above the chest. A reverse lordotic position is when the x-ray beam is pointed toward the feet.

NORMAL CHEST RADIOGRAPH

One of the most difficult aspects of evaluating the neonatal chest is the wide variation in the appearance of normal structures. The thymus, a lymphoid organ in the anterior mediastinum of neonates that plays an important role in immune system function, is a particular challenge.

In general, the thymus tends to have a wavy or undulating border, is less dense than the heart, and insinuates between or around structures rather than displacing them. The thymic border may be more apparent on the right or the left, but the thymus should always be centered in the anterior mediastinum. Because a prominent thymus can mimic cardiomegaly, a lateral view of the chest can help to clarify cardiac size.

Normal Thymic Borders

FIGURE 1-8

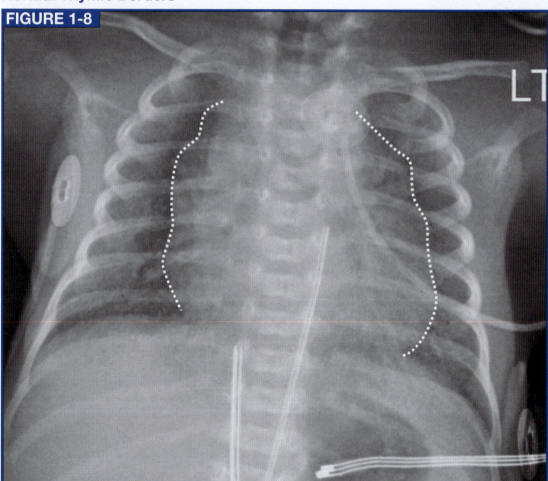

The prominent cardiomediastinal silhouette in this neonate is predominantly due to normal mediastinal thymic tissue, which demonstrates wavy borders and intermediate soft tissue density along the right and left mediastinal borders (dashed lines).

Normal Thymus Extended Toward the Right

FIGURE 1-9A

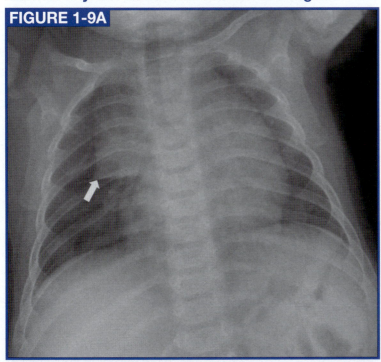

The normal thymus in this neonate is centered in the anterior mediastinum, but extends mostly toward the right (arrow).

FIGURE 1-9B

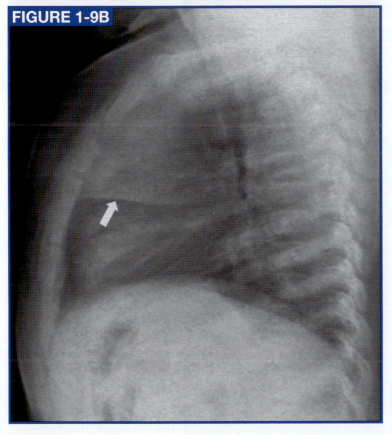

Note the thymic extension along the minor fissure, which creates a sharp inferior border (arrow).

Normal Thymus With Mass-Like Appearance

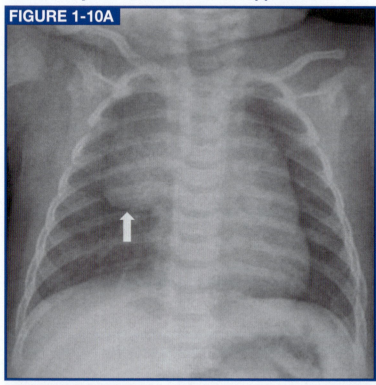

FIGURE 1-10A

This normal thymus has a more mass-like appearance (arrow).

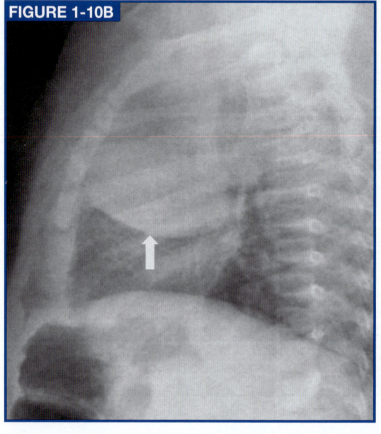

FIGURE 1-10B

The thymus extends along, but not below, the minor fissure (arrow).

Normal Thymus Extended Toward the Left

FIGURE 1-11

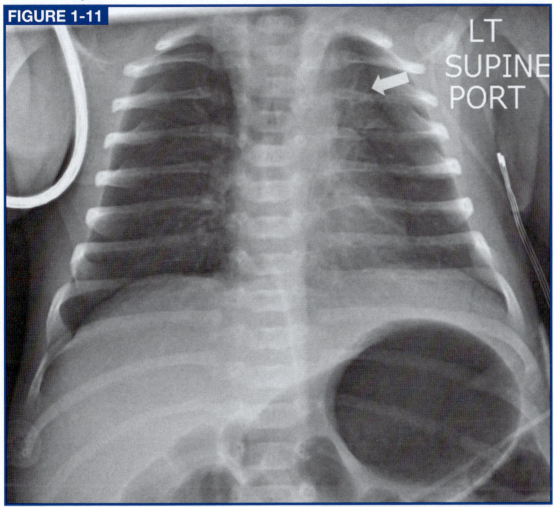

Normal thymic tissue in this neonate extends predominantly toward the left (arrow).

LUNG VOLUMES

Lung volumes are important to consider when managing patients with pulmonary or chest wall disease. A good way to estimate lung volume is to count the number of ribs that project over the lung spaces. Normally inflated lungs span approximately six anterior ribs, or eight to ten posterior ribs. In a well-positioned radiograph, the posterior ribs are longer and project horizontally, whereas the anterior ribs are shorter and curve at an angle. Note that the appearance of the ribs can change according to patient position and x-ray trajectory.

Small lung volumes are seen when the lungs are incompletely inflated. This hypoinflation crowds the interstitial structures, which manifests on chest radiographs as diffusely increased airspace opacity. This can mimic airspace diseases, such as pulmonary edema or infection.

Large lung volumes, or pulmonary hyperinflation, result in over-expanded airspaces, which manifest on chest radiographs as diffusely increased lucency. The diaphragm will appear flattened instead of having its normal domed shape.

Normal Lung Volumes

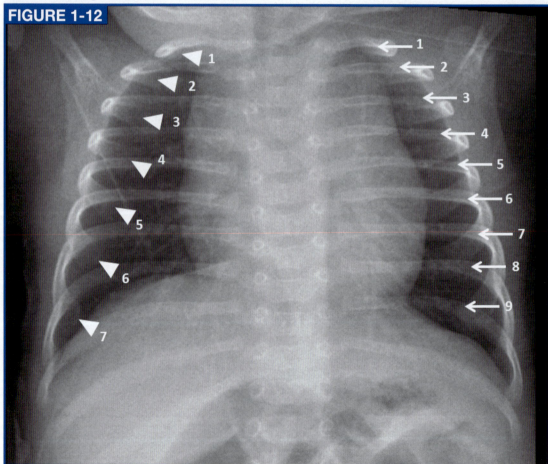

FIGURE 1-12

This chest radiograph demonstrates normal lung volumes, with the lungs spanning over six to seven anterior ribs (arrowheads) and nine posterior ribs (arrows).

Pulmonary Hypoinflation

FIGURE 1-13

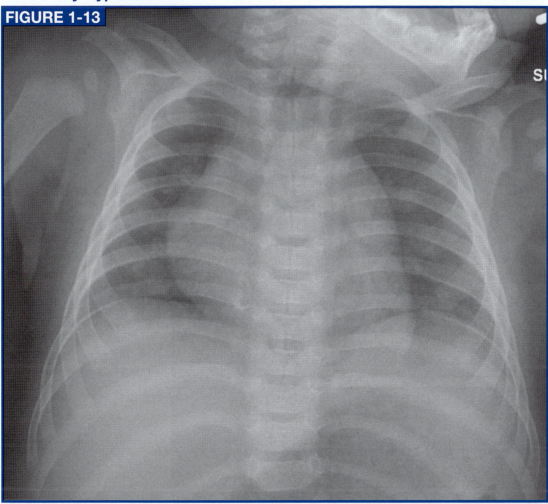

Here, small lung volumes and associated crowding of the interstitial structures create prominent interstitial markings and hazy opacification of the lungs, which can simulate disease.

Pulmonary Hyperinflation

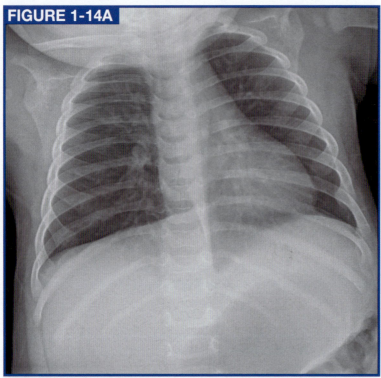

FIGURE 1-14A

In this example, large lung volumes create a generalized lucency of the lung. On the frontal view, the patient is slightly rotated toward the left.

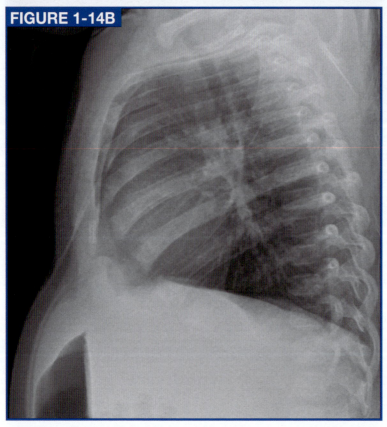

FIGURE 1-14B

Flattening of the hemidiaphragms relating to hyperinflation is better appreciated on the lateral view.

LINES AND TUBES
Endotracheal Tubes (ETTs)

The position of the head is an important consideration when evaluating the location of the ETT tip. Flexion of the neck will advance the tip toward the carina, while extension will displace it away from the carina. Head rotation to either side will draw the tip away from the carina.

Normal ETT Positioning

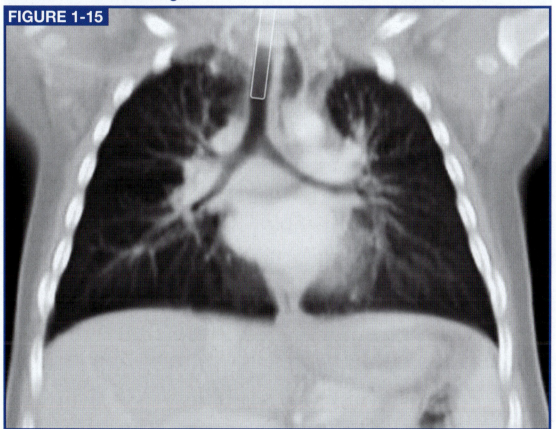

FIGURE 1-15

The tip of an appropriately positioned ETT is in the mid-thoracic trachea.

A tube positioned at or above the thoracic inlet may become dislodged. A tube too close to the carina may enter the right or left main bronchus, preventing ventilation to the contralateral lung.

Low ETT Positioning

FIGURE 1-16

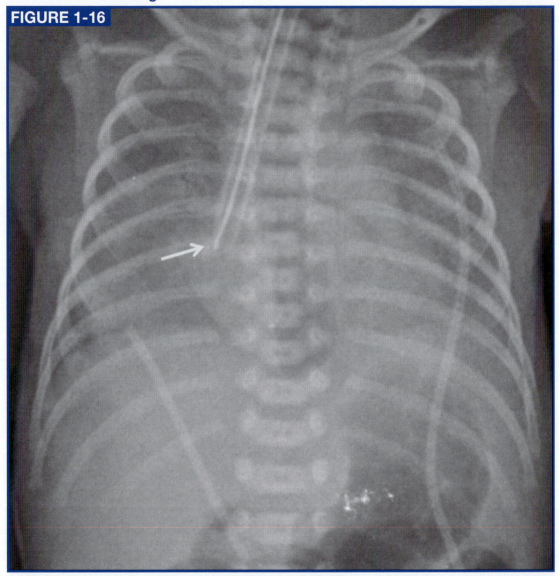

This ETT is too low, likely within the right lower-lobe bronchus, and needs to be repositioned (arrow).

Low ETT Positioning With Lung Collapse

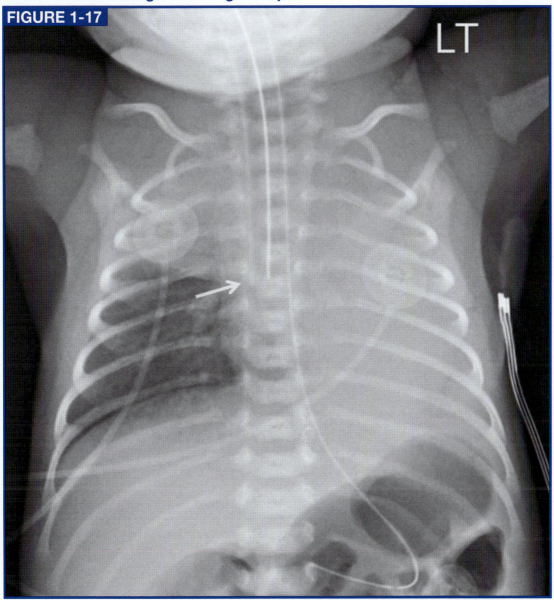

FIGURE 1-17

This tube is also positioned too low, likely in the bronchus intermedius (arrow). Collapse of the right upper lobe, left upper lobe, and left lower lobe has occurred due to inadequate ventilation. The tube requires immediate adjustment.

High ETT Positioning

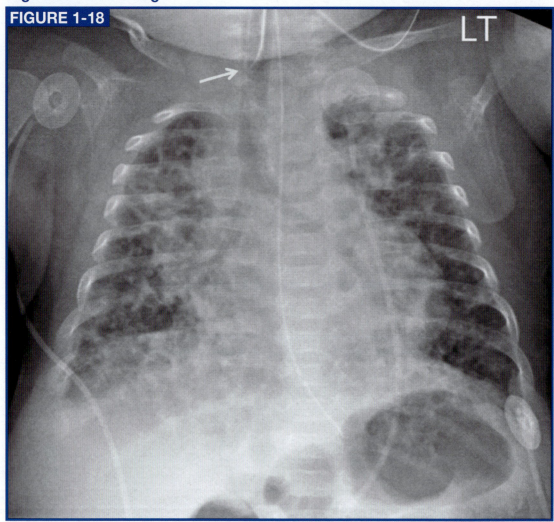

FIGURE 1-18

This ETT is positioned too high and projects above the thoracic inlet (arrow).

Peripherally Inserted Central Catheters (PICCs)

PICCs are used to administer fluids, medications, or nutrition, and can also be used for drawing blood. PICCs are most commonly placed in the upper extremities or the scalp and travel through the venous structures. The tip should be ideally positioned in the superior vena cava or at the superior cavoatrial junction. A lateral view may be helpful to evaluate course if positioning is unclear on the frontal view.

PICC Positioning in the Superior Vena Cava

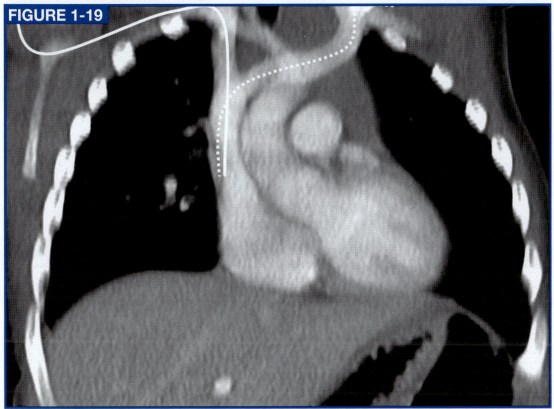

FIGURE 1-19

A PICC placed in the right upper extremity will travel through the right subclavian and right brachiocephalic veins into the superior vena cava (solid line). A PICC placed in the left upper extremity will travel through the left subclavian and left brachiocephalic veins into the superior vena cava (dashed line). A PICC placed in a scalp vein will travel through the jugular veins to the superior vena cava (not shown).

PICC Positioning at the Superior Cavoatrial Junction

FIGURE 1-20

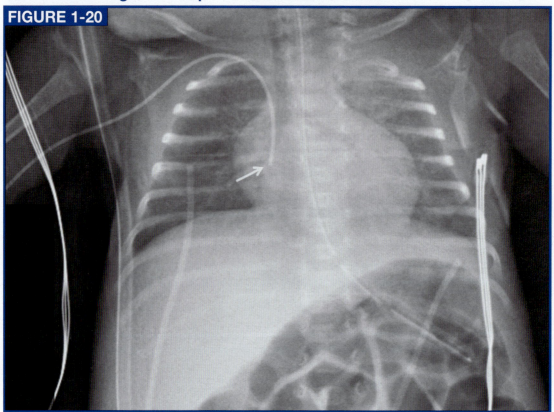

Placed in the right upper extremity, this PICC projects over the right axillary, right subclavian vein, and right brachiocephalic vein and terminates over the superior cavoatrial junction (arrow). The superior cavoatrial junction is located approximately two vertebral bodies below and to the right of the carina.

PICC Placement in the Left Scalp

FIGURE 1-21

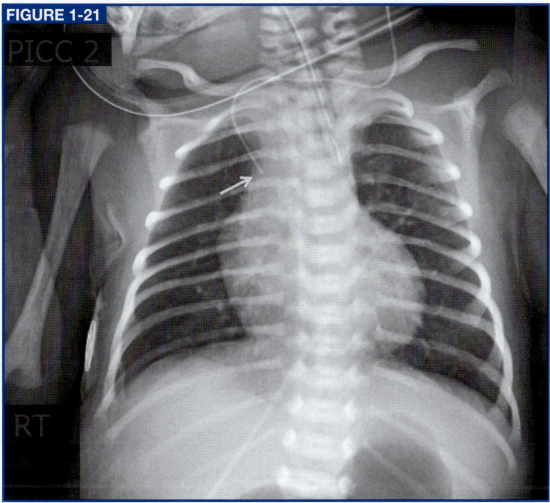

This PICC, which was placed in the left scalp, courses through the left internal jugular and left brachiocephalic veins. The tip is in ideal position over the superior vena cava (arrow).

PICC Showing Tributary Deviation

FIGURE 1-22

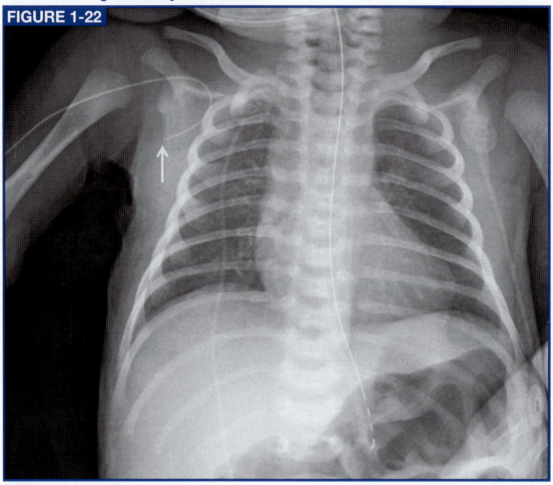

PICCs can deviate into small tributary venous structures and result in malpositioning. In this case, the PICC likely terminates in a small vein in the right axilla (arrow).

PICC With Cephalad Projection

FIGURE 1-23

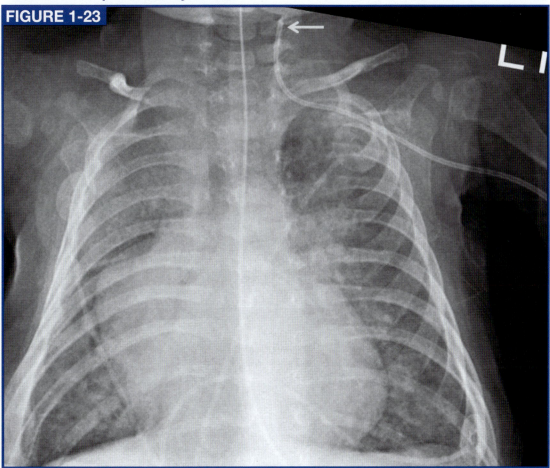

Upper extremity catheters can sometimes course cephalad into the jugular vein, as in this case (arrow), instead of inferiorly toward the superior vena cava.

PICC With Coiling

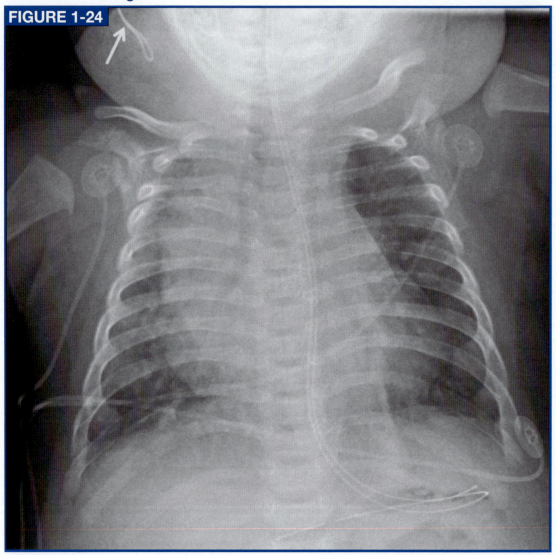

FIGURE 1-24

This right scalp PICC is coiled in the neck and needs to be repositioned (arrow).

PICC With Deviation Into Azygos Vein

FIGURE 1-25A

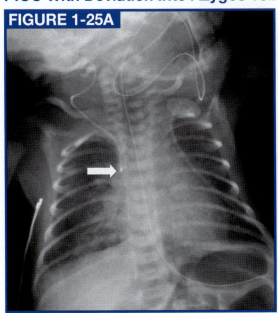

In this right scalp PICC placement, the catheter tip (arrow) appears to overlie the superior vena cava on the frontal view. Notice the increased density at the tip, however, which indicates that it is passing either anteriorly or posteriorly.

FIGURE 1-25B

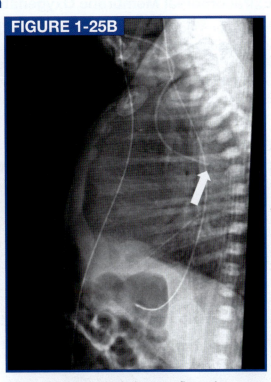

A cross-table lateral view confirms the posterior location of the PICC tip (arrow), likely within the azygos vein.

FIGURE 1-25C

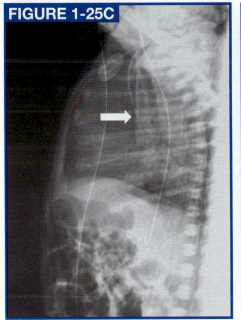

A second cross-table lateral view after 1.5 cm of withdrawal demonstrates that the PICC is in improved vertical orientation (arrow).

FIGURE 1-25D

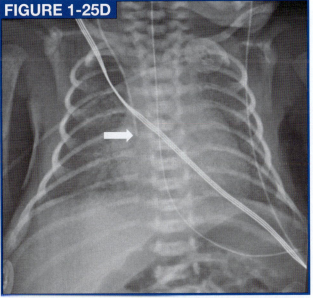

The final frontal radiograph demonstrates that the tip is in the appropriate position at the junction of the superior vena cava and the right atrium.

Extracorporeal Membrane Oxygenation (ECMO) Cannulae

ECMO provides blood-gas exchange outside the patient's body. It can be a life-saving intervention for critically ill neonates. Because they circulate large volumes of blood, ECMO cannulae are larger in caliber than other devices and are generally placed under the guidance of echocardiography. Blood exchange occurs via venovenous or venoarterial flow. The cannulae can be placed in a variety of positions within larger-sized vessels.

ECMO Cannula Positioning

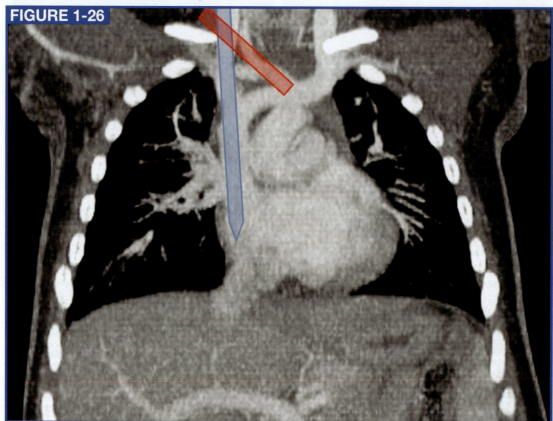

FIGURE 1-26

The ECMO cannulae are commonly placed through the neonate's internal jugular vein and superior vena cava for venous access (blue cannula), and through the carotid and innominate arteries for arterial access (red cannula). To avoid catastrophic hemorrhage, it is critical to ensure stable and adequate positioning of cannulae between studies.

Venovenous ECMO Placement

FIGURE 1-27

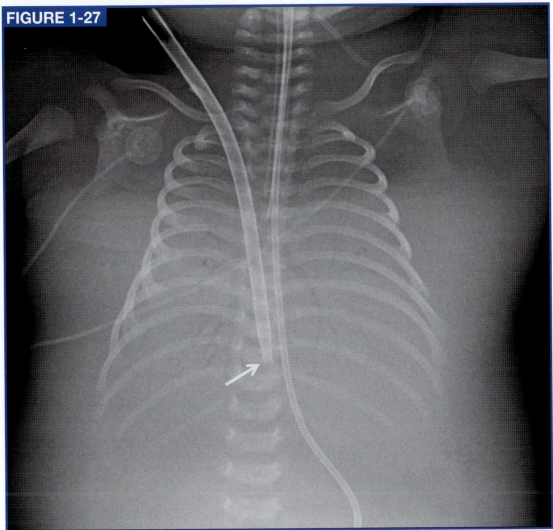

The tip of this venovenous ECMO cannula projects over the right atrium (arrow). The diffuse opacification of the lungs is an expected finding in a patient on ECMO. Chest wall edema is present, indicating third spacing.

Venoarterial ECMO Placement

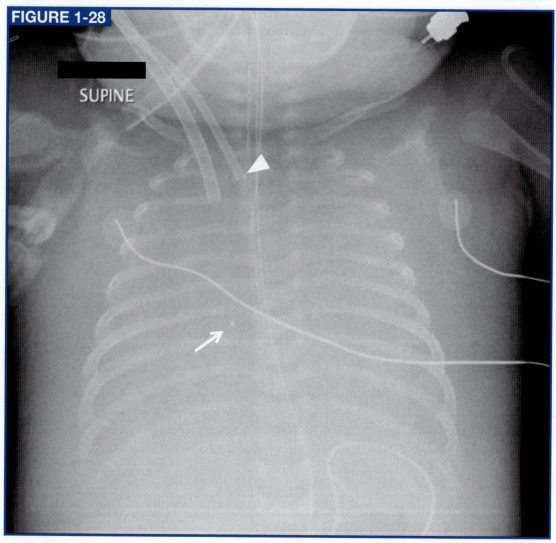

FIGURE 1-28

This image shows both venous and arterial cannulae. A radiopaque marker indicates the tip of the venous cannula over the region of the right atrium (arrow). The tip of the arterial cannula overlies the innominate artery (arrowhead).

THE PERIPHERY

While evaluation of cardiopulmonary structures is central to interpretation of neonatal chest radiographs, it is also important to consider structures outside of the cardiopulmonary system. The bones, upper abdomen, diaphragm, and subcutaneous tissues can provide essential information that impacts patient care.

Findings of Pneumatosis Intestinalis in the Periphery of the Chest Radiograph

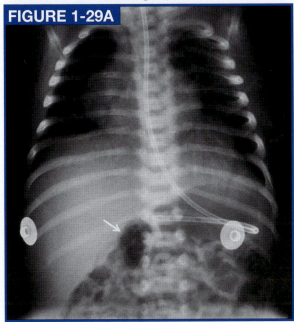

FIGURE 1-29A

After electronically adjusting the window and level of the chest radiograph, this 28-day-old infant with aortic coarctation was found to have pneumatosis intestinalis in the upper abdomen (arrow).

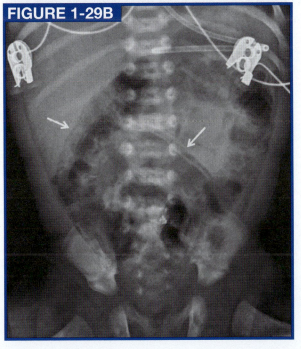

FIGURE 1-29B

On follow-up, an abdominal radiograph confirmed curvilinear lucencies along the bowel wall compatible with extensive pneumatosis throughout the abdomen (arrows).

Findings of Holt Oram Syndrome in the Periphery of the Chest Radiograph

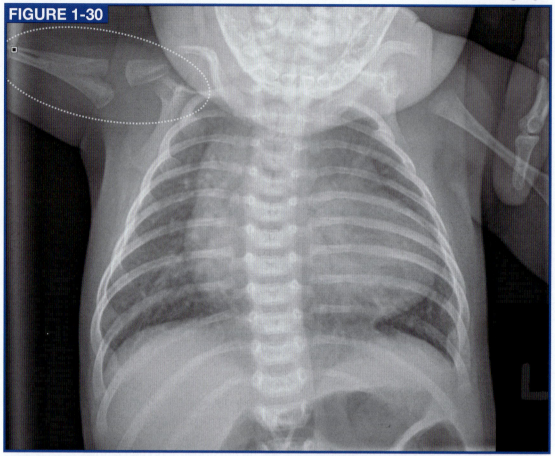

FIGURE 1-30

This initial chest radiograph in a patient with known congenital heart disease reveals right upper extremity deformity (dashed oval) compatible with a diagnosis of Holt Oram syndrome.

Hyperdensities in the Periphery of the Chest Radiograph

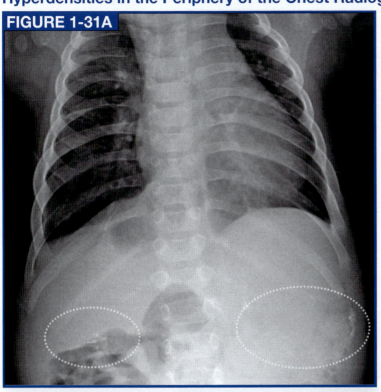
FIGURE 1-31A

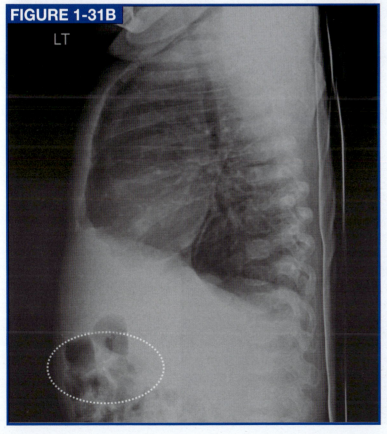
FIGURE 1-31B

Vague but persistent small hyperdensities were noted in the anterior upper abdomen (dashed ovals) on several studies of this neonate with a history of atrioventricular septal defect. These findings could indicate calcification from a prior episode of meconium peritonitis, partially calcified masses, or retained extravasated contrast material from a prior gastrointestinal leak.

Pneumoperitoneum in the Periphery of the Chest Radiograph

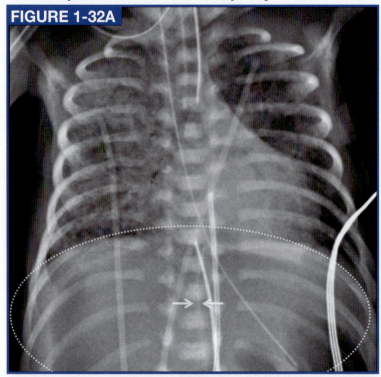

FIGURE 1-32A

This chest radiograph of an extremely low birth weight (ELBW) infant identified a large lucency in the upper abdomen (dashed oval) with an outline of the falciform ligament (arrows).

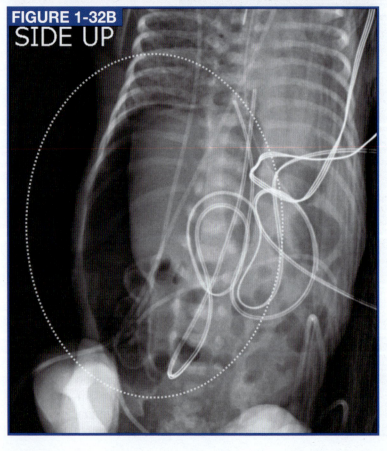

FIGURE 1-32B SIDE UP

The follow-up left-lateral decubitus view of the abdomen confirms a large-volume pneumoperitoneum (dashed oval).

PATHOLOGY
Pneumothorax

Imaging Findings

A pneumothorax appears as an abnormal lucency in the chest. Depending on location and patient positioning, it may manifest at the periphery of the thoracic cavity in association with a pleural line, or as vague lucency along the mediastinal border or lung base. An associated mediastinal shift to the contralateral side indicates tension pneumothorax, which requires emergent decompression.

Clinical Correlation

Pneumothoraces often occur in the presence of abnormal lung parenchyma, in association with positive-pressure ventilation (PPV), or as a result of increased intrathoracic pressures, such as during delivery. The patient may be tachypneic or hypoxic. Small pneumothoraces may be asymptomatic. Large pneumothoraces could rapidly progress to respiratory failure.

Key Points

- The Mach effect is an optical illusion that occurs between areas of different densities. On a chest radiograph, it often occurs at the mediastinal margin and can replicate a pneumothorax or pneumomediastinum. This entity is discussed further in Chapter 5.

- Follow-up imaging in the decubitus position may better demonstrate the suspected pneumothorax and the pleural line.

Pneumothorax With Pleural Line

FIGURE 1-33

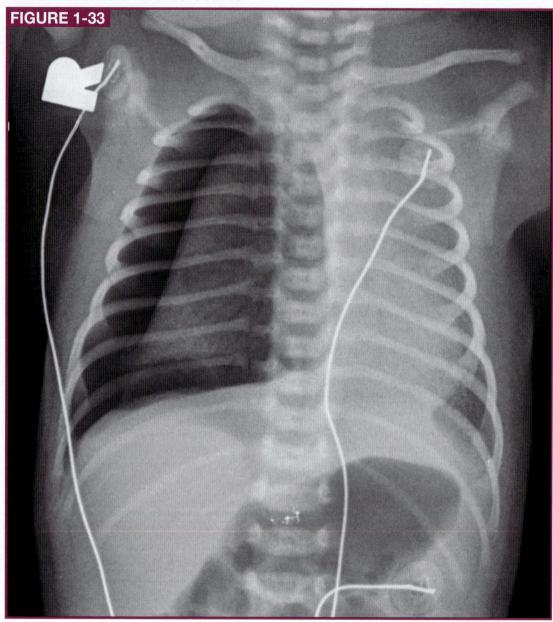

This image shows a large right-sided pneumothorax in which the lung markings do not extend to the lateral ribs and the pleural line is obvious. The mediastinum is deviated into the non-rotated patient's left chest, which is compatible with tension pneumothorax.

Pneumothorax With Near-Complete Resolution

FIGURE 1-34

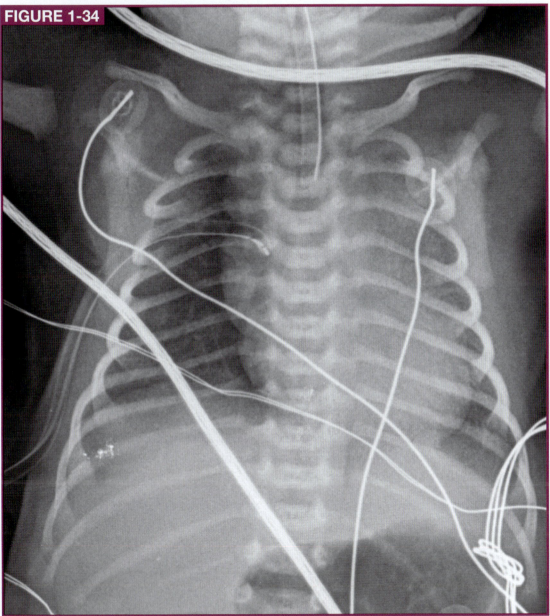

This follow-up radiograph obtained after chest tube placement reveals near-complete resolution of the right-sided pneumothorax. Residual lucency along the right cardiac border indicates a small residual anteromedial pneumothorax. The patient had been intubated since the prior study.

Pneumothorax With Pulmonary Hypoplasia

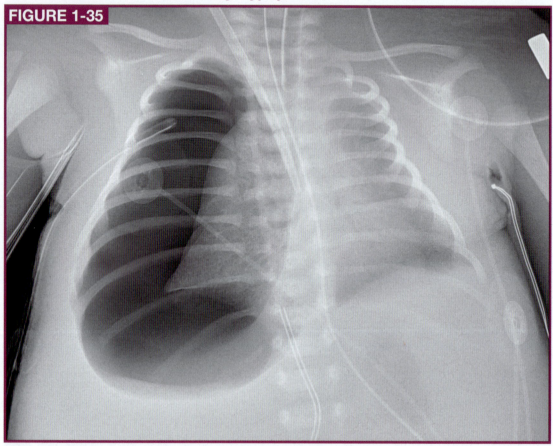

FIGURE 1-35

Another example of tension pneumothorax in a patient on ECMO. The patient had end-stage renal disease with pulmonary hypoplasia at birth.

Pneumothorax With Deep Costophrenic Sulcus Sign

FIGURE 1-36

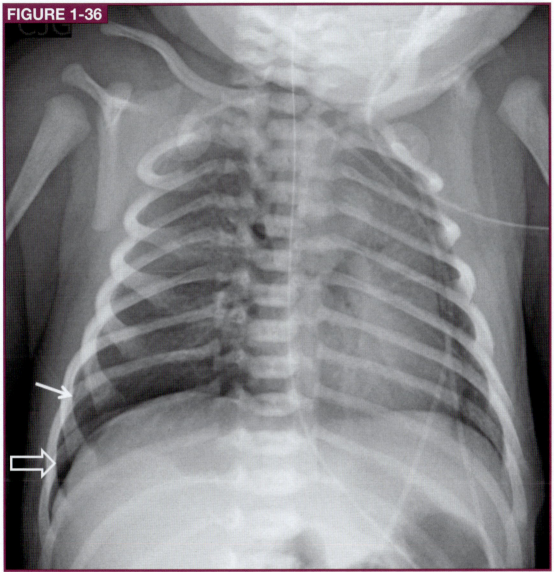

This small pneumothorax is barely visible at the right costophrenic angle (arrow). Generalized lucency at the lung base, in combination with an asymmetrically deep costophrenic sulcus, sometimes referred to as the "deep costophrenic sulcus sign" (open arrow), support the diagnosis. The patient is considerably rotated toward the left.

Pneumothorax With Decubitus View

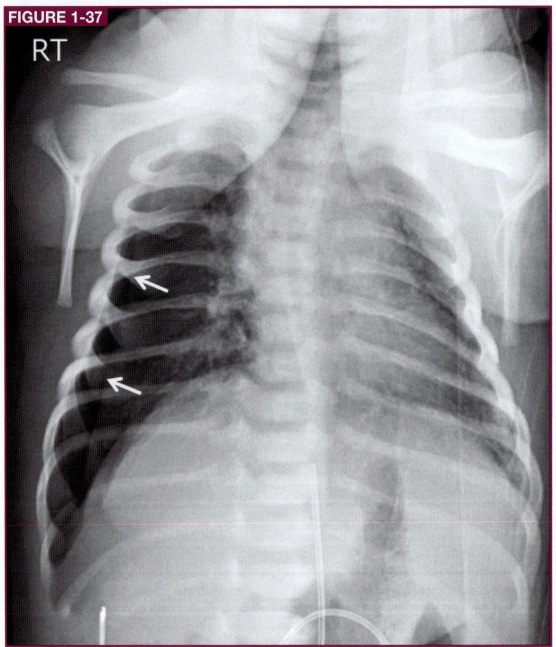

FIGURE 1-37

This small right-sided pneumothorax (arrows) is best demonstrated with a left-lateral decubitus view, in which the patient's left side is positioned on the bed or table. In the decubitus view, the side of suspected pneumothorax should be directed away from the table so that pleural cavity gas can collect in the nondependent portion of the chest, where it is seen more clearly.

Pneumomediastinum

Imaging Findings

Pneumomediastinum appears as abnormal lucency in or along the mediastinum. It often lifts or displaces the thymus, creating a characteristic appearance in the neonate referred to as the "spinnaker-sail sign." Localization of pneumomediastinum may be improved with a cross-table lateral view. A lateral decubitus view can be helpful to differentiate pneumomediastinum from pneumothorax in difficult cases.

Clinical Correlation

Pneumomediastinum may be associated with PPV and barotrauma, as a result of surgery or percutaneous procedures, or it may be idiopathic. Anterior pneumomediastinum often resolves on its own without intervention. Posterior pneumomediastinum can be serious, leading to impaired return of oxygenated blood to the heart and tamponade physiology.

Key Points

- Pneumomediastinum may extend along fascial planes to multiple anatomic structures, including the pleural space, retropharyngeal space, vascular sheaths in the neck, and retroperitoneal space in the upper abdomen. Gas extension into these areas is not uncommon and can be observed by radiograph.

- Careful clinical observation and radiographic follow-up are often all that is required for anterior pneumomediastinum, which, in isolation, generally has a benign course.

Pneumomediastinum With Spinnaker-Sail Sign

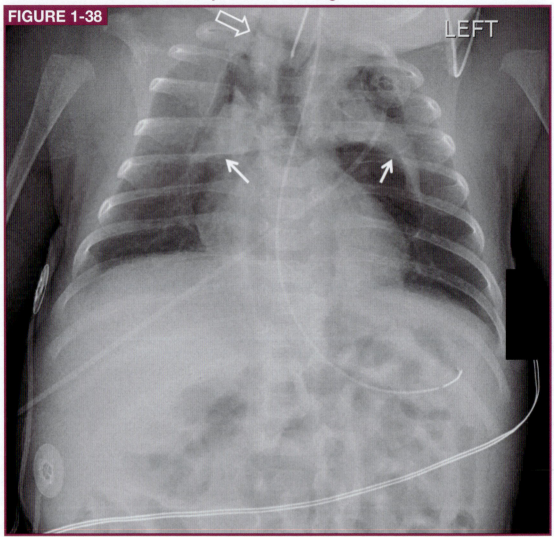

FIGURE 1-38

This extensive pneumomediastinum shows the characteristic spinnaker-sail appearance of the thymus (arrows). Gas is also seen dissecting along the vascular sheaths into the neck (open arrow).

Anterior Pneumomediastinum

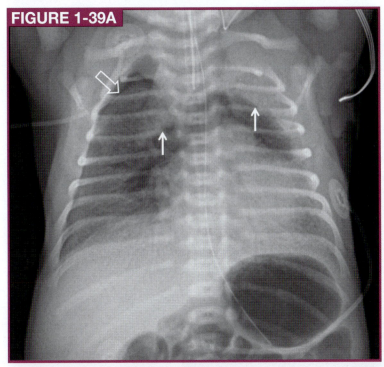

FIGURE 1-39A

Frontal view of the chest in a different patient with pneumomediastinum shows lucency outlining the thymic tissue (arrows) with a small right pneumothorax (open arrow).

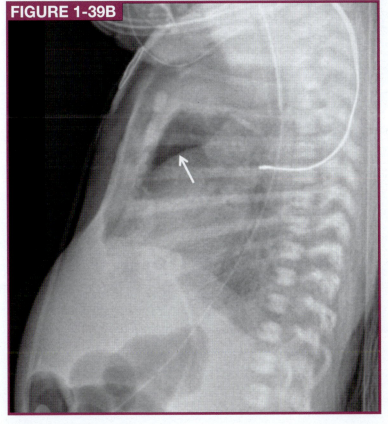

FIGURE 1-39B

Cross-table lateral view shows lucency in the anterior mediastinum.

Pulmonary Interstitial Emphysema (PIE)

Imaging Findings

PIE most commonly appears as linear branching lucencies that follow the bronchovascular bundles. The lucencies represent collections of gas that have leaked out of the airway. Findings can be diffuse, asymmetric, or focal and may progress to pneumothorax or pneumomediastinum.

Clinical Correlation

PIE occurs in neonates with lung diseases such as surfactant deficiency, meconium aspiration syndrome, or infection. It is often associated with PPV, but can also occur in extremely premature infants with low mean airway pressure ventilation.

Key Points

- Patients with PIE require intensive respiratory management to reduce morbidity and mortality. Suspicious radiographic findings should not be overlooked.

PIE Patterns

These radiographs show different patterns of PIE in three different patients.

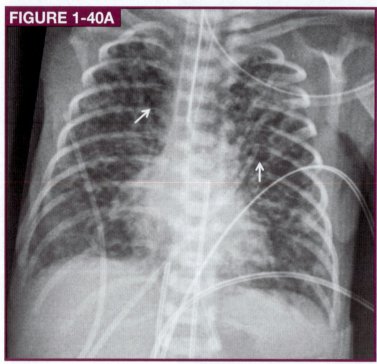

FIGURE 1-40A

Diffuse pattern of PIE is demonstrated, with symmetric branching lucencies extending from the hila (arrows).

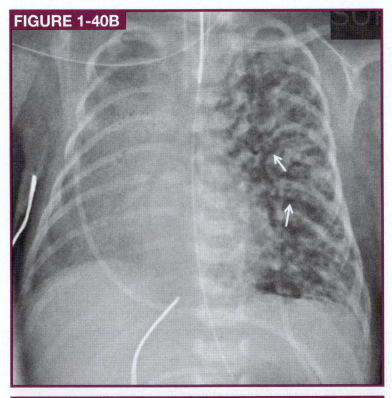

FIGURE 1-40B

Unilateral left-sided PIE pattern is present (arrows).

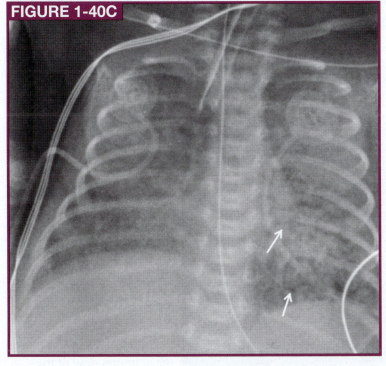

FIGURE 1-40C

Focal PIE of the left lower lobe (arrows).

Atelectasis

Imaging Findings

Atelectasis manifests as a focal density in the lung due to lung collapse. Affected areas range from small linear or patchy subsegmental portions to an entire lobe or lung. A key imaging feature is volume loss as the gas leaves the airways and alveolar spaces and the lung interstitium consolidates.

Clinical Correlation

Atelectasis is an extremely common finding in the neonatal chest, due to a combination of the collapsible nature of the neonatal airway, the small airway size, and the frequency of pulmonary disease that leads to airway blockage. Atelectasis can also be iatrogenic, as occurs with malpositioning of an ETT. Patients may be hypoxic, particularly if larger areas of lung are involved.

Key Points

- Rapid changes in a focal opacity — for example, an opacity that appears or resolves within 24 hours — is more common with atelectasis than with infection or hemorrhage.

- Both volume-positive processes, such as pleural effusion, hemorrhage, or neoplasm; and volume-negative processes, such as atelectasis; can cause "white out" of an entire lung. Atelectasis and volume loss are indicated by a shift of the mediastinum, fissure, or diaphragm toward the opacified lung.

Migrating Atelectasis

Three sequential chest radiographs, obtained within 24 hours, reveal migrating areas of atelectasis (dashed circles) in an infant with lung disease of prematurity.

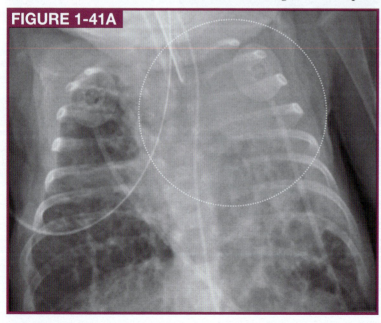

FIGURE 1-41A

Initial frontal view of the chest reveals dense left upper-lobe atelectasis with leftward mediastinal shift.

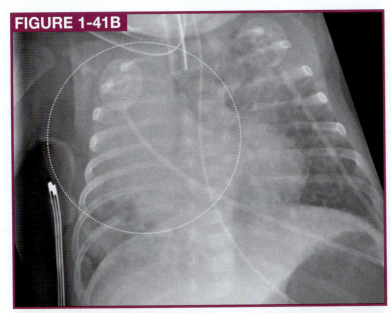

FIGURE 1-41B

Repeat imaging obtained several hours later demonstrates improved aeration of the left upper lobe with new dense right upper-lobe atelectasis and rightward mediastinal shift.

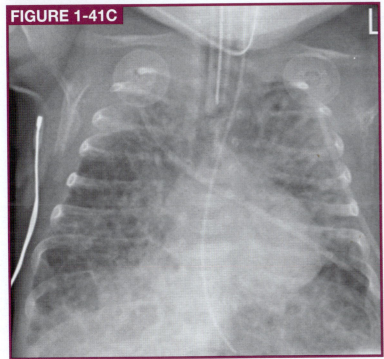

FIGURE 1-41C

Another study obtained a few hours later shows that the lower lobes are better aerated and there is only mild patchy atelectasis in the upper lobes. The mediastinum is normally located.

Surfactant Deficiency

Imaging Findings

Premature infants frequently have surfactant deficiency in the lungs due to inadequate surfactant production by pneumatocytes. Imaging findings include diffuse granular interstitial lung densities, which resemble tiny dots sprinkled over the lung tissue, and a generalized haziness due to capillary leakage. Lung volumes are usually decreased and air bronchograms are common.

Clinical Correlation

Respiratory distress syndrome (RDS) is the clinical term associated with neonatal surfactant deficiency. Neonates with RDS typically present with tachypnea, grunting, nasal flaring, cyanosis, and substernal and intercostal retractions. Administration of maternal steroids prenatally has been shown to decrease the incidence of RDS and is often performed if preterm delivery is anticipated.

Key Points

- While surfactant deficiency is usually a diffuse process, intratracheal administration of surfactant replacement agents can lead to asymmetric findings of surfactant deficiency and lung aeration.

- Prematurity is cited as the cause of surfactant deficiency in a vast majority of cases. However, a small percentage may be due to genetic defects that prevent the normal formation of surfactant.

Examples of Surfactant Deficiency

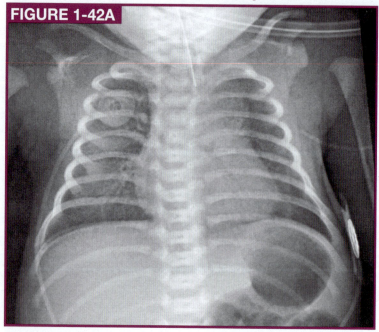

FIGURE 1-42A Mild diffuse changes of surfactant deficiency are demonstrated, including scattered granular interstitial densities and hazy lung opacities.

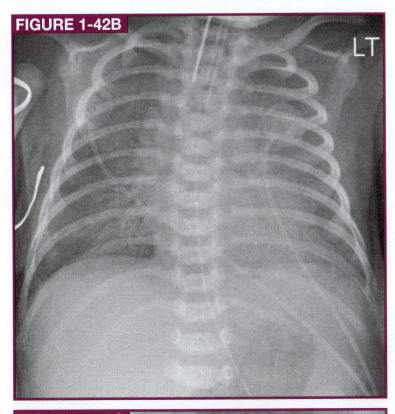

FIGURE 1-42B

The findings of surfactant deficiency in another preterm patient are moderately severe.

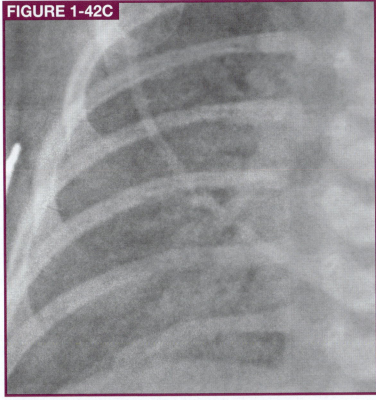

FIGURE 1-42C

The diffuse granular opacities (tiny dots) and air bronchograms (central branching lucencies) from the patient in Fig. B are better demonstrated in this magnified image.

Bronchopulmonary Dysplasia (BPD)

Imaging Findings

BPD appears as coarse interstitial markings, often with scattered small cystic lucencies. Pulmonary hyperinflation is commonly associated.

Clinical Correlation

BPD is characterized by abnormal respiratory function in premature infants who require supplemental oxygen for at least 28 days after birth. The definition and diagnosis of BPD have changed over time. Infants born after 32 weeks gestational age now have milder long-term radiographic and clinical manifestations than those from decades past. Changes of BPD are now detected prior to 28 days of life in very low birth weight (VLBW) and ELBW infants. Mild, moderate, and severe BPD are defined by physiologic criteria, such as degree of oxygen requirement and need for PPV at 36 weeks postmenstrual age, rather than by radiographic findings.

Key Points

- Patients with BPD, who often require PPV for adequate oxygenation, should be closely evaluated for evidence of pneumothorax and pneumomediastinum.

Examples of BPD

FIGURE 1-43A

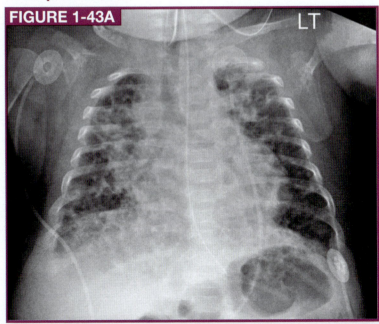

Frontal radiograph of an infant with BPD shows thick interstitial markings and scattered cystic lucencies bilaterally throughout the lungs. The lungs are hyperinflated, a common associated finding, and there is superimposed subsegmental atelectasis in both upper lobes, as well as in the right lower lobe. The patient is intubated due to respiratory failure. Note the high position of the ETT tip, which was subsequently repositioned.

FIGURE 1-43B

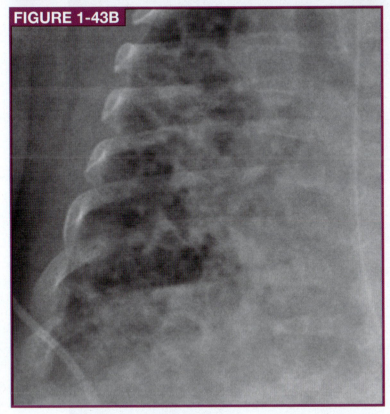

A magnified view of the same patient better demonstrates the thick interstitial markings and cystic lucencies of BPD.

Pulmonary Hemorrhage

Imaging Findings

Pulmonary hemorrhage most commonly manifests as extensive, diffuse airspace opacities throughout the lungs, but can also present with focal or asymmetric findings. Air bronchograms are usually present.

Clinical Correlation

Fresh blood coming from the ETT or trachea raises clinical suspicion for pulmonary hemorrhage. The exact etiology is unknown, but pulmonary hemorrhage can occur in premature infants and often correlates with a deteriorating clinical course.

Key Points

- The imaging appearance of pulmonary hemorrhage is nonspecific and must be correlated with the clinical course.

Example of Pulmonary Hemorrhage

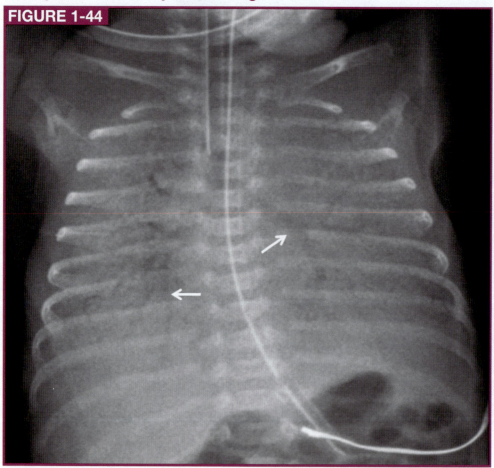

FIGURE 1-44

This premature infant with pulmonary hemorrhage shows diffuse opacities throughout the lungs. Air bronchograms are present bilaterally (arrows).

Transient Tachypnea of the Newborn

Imaging Findings

Diffuse, fine interstitial opacities, small pleural effusions, and normal lung volumes are hallmarks of transient tachypnea of the newborn. ETTs are not needed for these patients because they do not progress to respiratory failure. Findings typically resolve or improve significantly by 24 hours of life if repeat imaging is obtained.

Clinical Correlation

The lungs fill with amniotic fluid prenatally, which is quickly exchanged for air in the immediate postnatal period. If pulmonary fluid is not completely eliminated from the lungs, retained fetal fluid leads to transient tachypnea of the newborn. Supportive treatment with oxygen, intravenous fluids, and gavage feeds are usually all that is needed until the fluid is resorbed and the tachypnea resolves.

Key Points

- Transient tachypnea of the newborn occurs more commonly in patients born via caesarian section, which does not allow for the normal compression of the thoracic cavity that occurs with vaginal delivery.

- Small pleural effusions are subtle in infants, but upon close inspection, linear opacities can be seen tracking along the lateral chest wall near the costophrenic angle.

Example of Transient Tachypnea of the Newborn

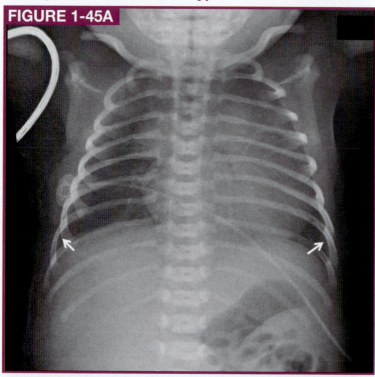

FIGURE 1-45A Fine interstitial opacities and very small pleural effusions (arrows) are seen in a patient with transient tachypnea of the newborn. Note the prominent size of the cardiomediastinal silhouette due to thymic tissue.

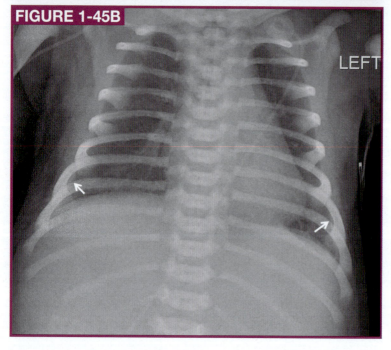

FIGURE 1-45B Similar fine interstitial densities and small pleural effusions (arrows) are present in a second infant with transient tachypnea of the newborn.

Neonatal Pneumonia

Imaging Findings

Imaging findings of neonatal pneumonia are variable and nonspecific. They may include reticulonodular opacities, patchy airspace opacities, pulmonary hyperinflation, and pleural effusions.

Clinical Correlation

Because the imaging appearance is inconsistent, clinical presentation is key to diagnosis. Pneumonia is the most frequent cause of septicemia in a neonate. Group B *Streptococcus* is the most common organism associated with pneumonia in the first week of life.

Key Points

- Neonatal pneumonia occurs within the first 28 days of life. It can be caused by infection *in utero*, during delivery, or in the first four weeks after birth.

- The infant should be carefully evaluated for pneumothorax, pneumomediastinum, and pneumatoceles, which occur as complications of neonatal pneumonia.

Example of Neonatal Pneumonia

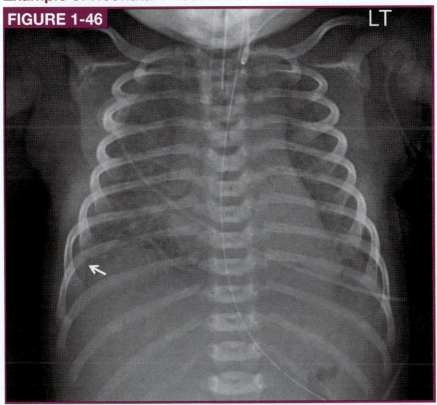

FIGURE 1-46

This infant with neonatal pneumonia has diffuse interstitial densities, patchy opacities throughout the right lung, and a small right pleural effusion. An ETT is in place due to respiratory failure.

Meconium Aspiration Syndrome

Imaging Findings

Coarse and ropey lung markings, patchy consolidations, and pulmonary hyperinflation are radiographic hallmarks of meconium aspiration syndrome. Pleural effusions may also be seen in a subset of patients. An ETT is often present, indicating progression to respiratory failure.

Clinical Correlation

A clinical history of meconium-stained amniotic fluid at birth and respiratory distress or failure should raise the suspicion of meconium aspiration syndrome. The severity of illness varies widely. Some neonates require ECMO for profound hypoxemia in the setting of pulmonary disease.

Key Points

- Filling of the bronchi with meconium can lead to a ball-valve effect that prevents complete expiration of air. This leads to air trapping and contributes to pulmonary hyperinflation.

- Given the ball-valve effect of meconium, infants with meconium aspiration syndrome are at increased risk for pneumomediastinum and pneumothorax.

Meconium Aspiration Syndrome With Pulmonary Hyperinflation

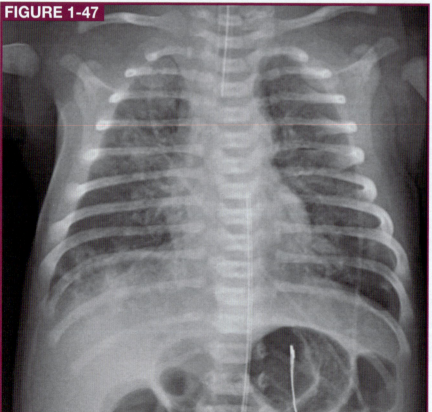

FIGURE 1-47 Coarse lung markings and patchy opacities are seen throughout the lungs in this intubated patient with meconium aspiration syndrome. Eight anterior ribs project over the lungs bilaterally, indicating pulmonary hyperinflation.

Congenital Heart Disease (CHD)

Imaging Findings

There are wide variations in the imaging appearance of CHD in neonates. Often, a congenital heart defect is already suspected based on prenatal imaging. In other cases, cardiomegaly, abnormal pulmonary vasculature, abnormal mediastinal contours, or pulmonary edema on radiography serve as clues. Ultimately, cross-sectional imaging with echocardiogram, CT, or MRI is needed to fully characterize abnormalities of cardiac anatomy and function.

Clinical Correlation

Infants with CHD may present with difficulty in breathing, cyanosis, feeding intolerance, poor weight gain, or body swelling. A murmur is sometimes detected on physical exam. Severity of disease ranges broadly. Some patients are critically ill from birth, while minor defects may not be detected until adulthood.

Key Points

- A lateral view may be helpful to evaluate heart size if cardiomegaly is suspected on a frontal view. Although thymic tissue will always project in the anterior mediastinum in a lateral view, true heart enlargement is indicated by abnormal posterior extension of the cardiac border.

- Chest radiographs help determine the presence of or changes in pulmonary edema in patients being treated for CHD. It may manifest as increased interstitial markings or hazy airspace opacities and is typically symmetric in distribution, often with associated pleural effusions.

Pulmonary Edema

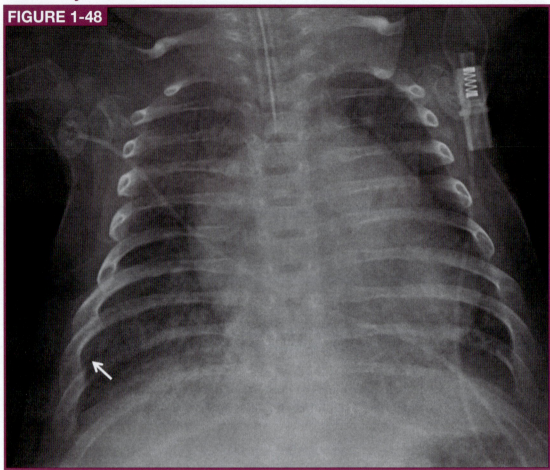

FIGURE 1-48

A patient with atrioventricular septal defect has cardiomegaly and diffusely increased interstitial markings compatible with pulmonary edema. A small right pleural effusion is present (arrow). Patchy densities in the right upper and lower lobe likely represent superimposed atelectasis.

Hypoplastic Left Heart Syndrome

FIGURE 1-49

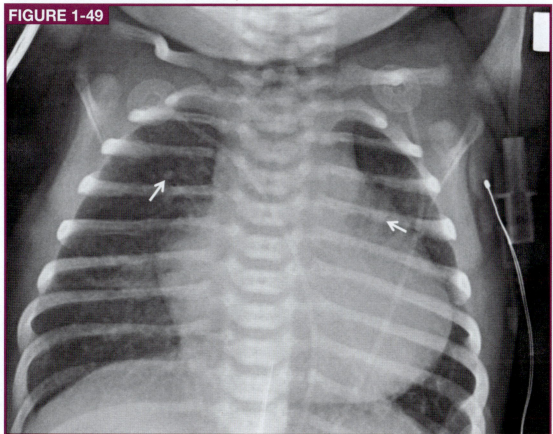

The heart is enlarged and demonstrates abnormal contour in this patient with hypoplastic left heart syndrome. There are increased vascular markings centrally (arrows) and mild edema is present.

Tetralogy of Fallot

FIGURE 1-50

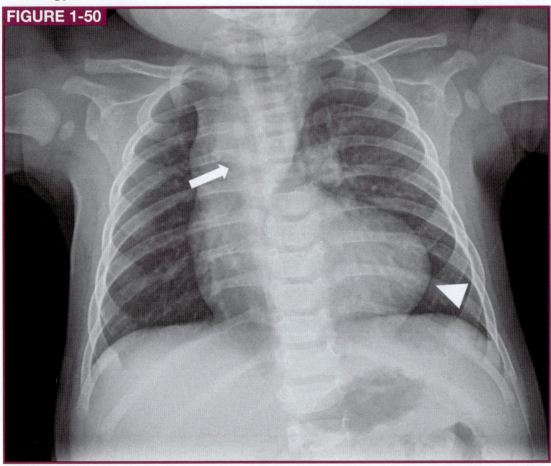

This patient with Tetralogy of Fallot demonstrates classic abnormal upturning of the cardiac apex (arrowhead). The patient also has a right-sided aortic arch, which is seen here as a vertically oriented, right paravertebral density (arrow). There is a higher incidence of right-sided aortic arch in patients with this type of congenital heart defect.

Congenital Diaphragmatic Hernia (CDH)

Imaging Findings

The two radiographic findings with highest specificity for CDH are the presence of gas-filled bowel loops in the chest and deviation of an enteric tube into the chest. These indicate that abdominal contents have herniated into the thoracic cavity through a diaphragmatic defect.

Clinical Correlation

Most neonates with CDH are very ill at birth due to pulmonary hypoplasia that occurs when the abdominal contents fill the chest. ECMO may be required as a bridge to surgery in the postnatal period.

Key Points

- Decompressed intrathoracic bowel loops without intraluminal gas can be mistaken for other types of cardiopulmonary disease. Carefully evaluate for evidence of contralateral mediastinal shift and other signs of diaphragmatic hernia in these instances. Gas-filled intrathoracic bowel loops can also mimic cystic lung masses. A chest ultrasound may help identify peristalsing intrathoracic bowel loops in unclear cases.

- CDH occurs more commonly on the left side than on the right. Bilateral cases are rare.

Bochdalek CDH Opening on the Left Side of the Diaphragm

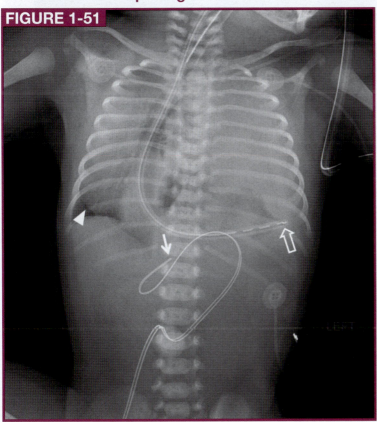

FIGURE 1-51

This image demonstrates a large left-sided posterior (Bochdalek) diaphragmatic hernia. The bowel is predominantly decompressed, with soft tissue density filling the left chest. There is associated rightward mediastinal shift (arrowhead). The enteric tube (open arrow) and umbilical venous catheter (arrow) have an abnormal course.

CDH With Partially Gas-Filled Bowel Loops

FIGURE 1-52

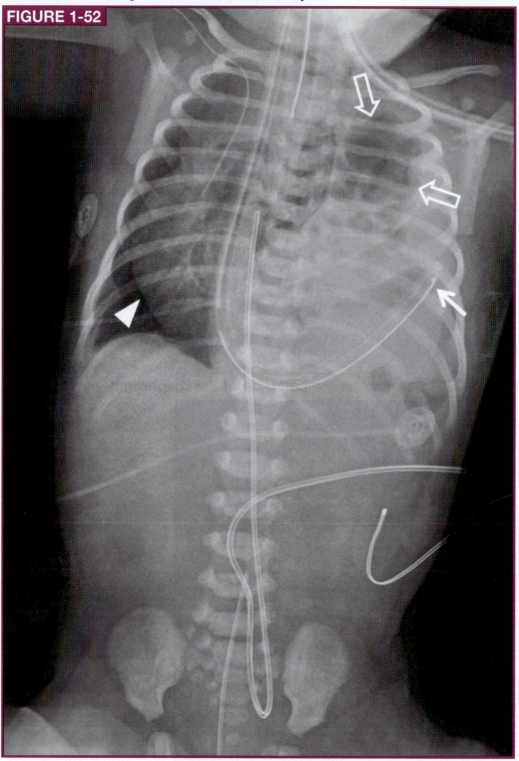

This CDH patient's intrathoracic bowel loops are partially gas filled (open arrows). The intrathoracic position of the stomach has caused the enteric tube to deviate into the chest (arrow). Rightward mediastinal shift is present (arrowhead).

CDH Obtained on Fetal MRI

FIGURE 1-53

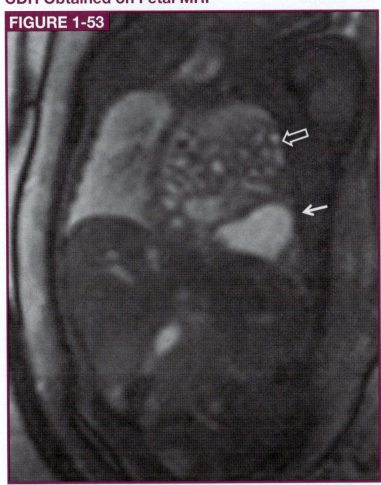

In a similar case, fetal MRI shows a left-sided CDH that contains the patient's stomach (arrow) and bowel (open arrow). Fetal lung volumes can be calculated from the MRI study to obtain prognostic information in the prenatal period.

CDH With Gas-Filled Bowel Loops

FIGURE 1-54

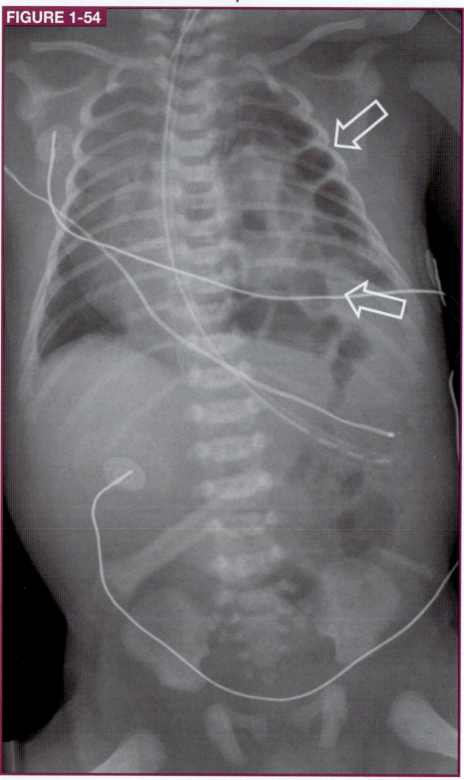

This chest and abdomen radiograph in another neonate with a left-sided CDH shows gas-filled bowel loops in the left chest (open arrows). The stomach is intra-abdominal.

CDH With Anterior Diaphragmatic Defect

This is a rare type of CDH, either retrosternal or parasternal.

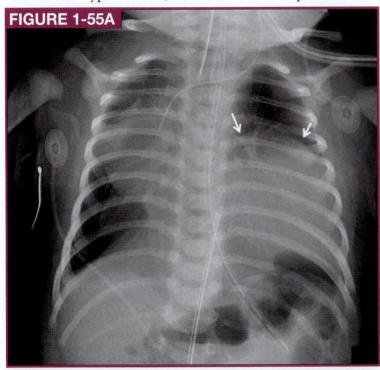

An anterior (Morgagni) CDH, which includes the patient's liver (arrows), is shown on chest radiograph.

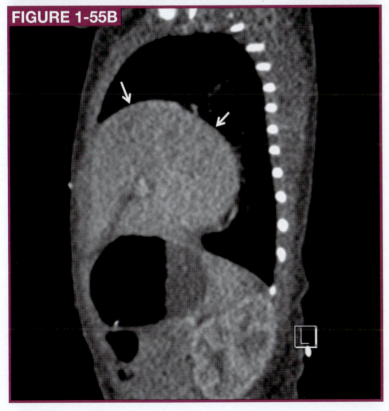

A sagittal image from the corresponding chest CT shows the liver clearly herniating into the chest anteriorly (arrows).

Congenital Pulmonary Airway Malformation (CPAM)

Imaging Findings

CPAM manifests as an abnormal cystic or solid area in any lobe of the lung. Small lesions may be radiographically subtle or occult. Large lesions can cause mediastinal shift. CT is often used in the first year of life to provide superior anatomic characterization in preparation for surgical resection.

Clinical Correlation

CPAM results from focal abnormal lung development. Patients with a CPAM lesion may be asymptomatic, or could have significant respiratory distress or failure. The clinical course predominantly depends on the size of the lesion.

Key Points

- CPAMs vary in appearance from macrocystic to microcystic to solid. They often coexist with pulmonary sequestration, forming hybrid lesions.

- Prenatal diagnosis of CPAM is increasing as the use of high-quality prenatal imaging rises. Fetal MRI may be performed to characterize these lung masses and provide prognostic information. Mothers of infants suspected to have large CPAM lesions may be encouraged to deliver at a tertiary care center with NICU and pediatric surgical services.

- Surgical resection is often performed due to an increased risk of recurrent infection and a small association with malignancy.

CPAM on Radiograph

FIGURE 1-56

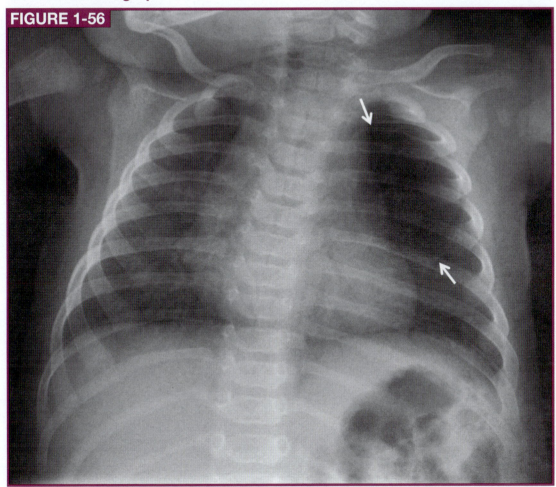

This radiograph shows a large cystic mass in the left upper lobe, compatible with CPAM (arrows).

CPAM on Follow-Up CT

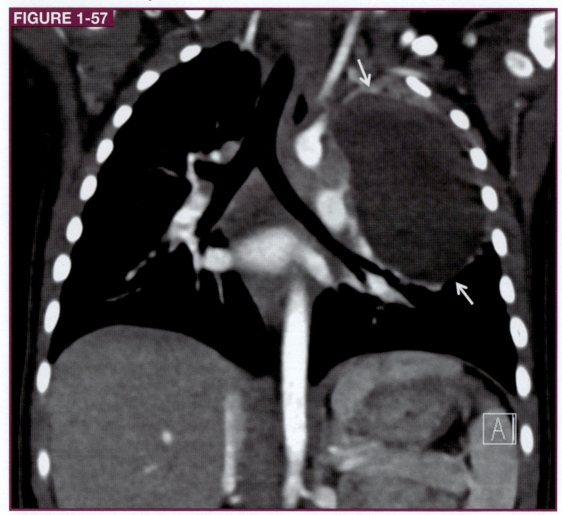

FIGURE 1-57

A subsequent CT scan of the same patient reveals a unilocular cyst that has filled with fluid since the prior radiograph (arrows). This could indicate superinfection of the lesion in the interim.

Pulmonary Sequestration

Imaging Findings

A persistent solid opacity in the lower lobe of a neonate should raise suspicion for pulmonary sequestration. Pulmonary sequestration is associated with anomalous systemic arterial supply and venous drainage. The area of abnormal lung does not communicate with the bronchial tree or pulmonary arteries, which is best demonstrated on advanced imaging such as CT angiogram.

Clinical Correlation

Patients with pulmonary sequestration may present with respiratory distress. It is not uncommon for patients to present later in life with chronic cough or recurrent infections in the lower lobe of the lung. Surgical resection is almost always pursued.

Key Points

- Pulmonary sequestration often coexists with CPAM, forming hybrid lesions.

- Similar to CPAM, prenatal diagnosis of sequestration is increasing with the frequent use of high-quality prenatal imaging. Fetal MRI may be performed to characterize these lung masses and provide prognostic information.

Pulmonary Sequestration on Radiograph and CT

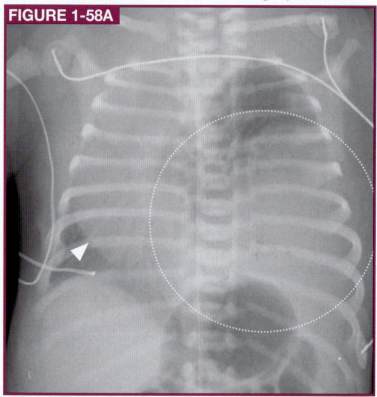

FIGURE 1-58A

This chest radiograph demonstrates a large left-sided mass centered in the neonate's left lower lobe (dashed circle) with associated rightward deviation of the mediastinal structures (arrowhead).

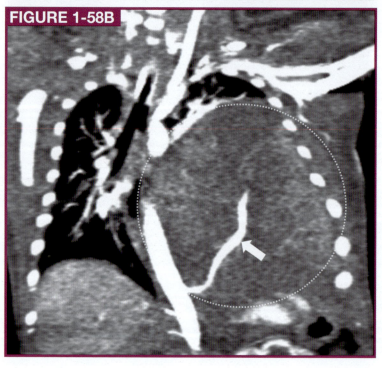

FIGURE 1-58B

A CT angiogram from the same patient shows an anomalous artery extending from the descending thoracic aorta (arrow) to supply the lesion (dashed circle), which is compatible with a large pulmonary sequestration.

Pulmonary Sequestration on MRI and Radiograph

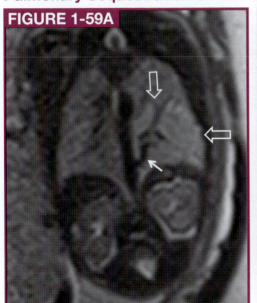

FIGURE 1-59A

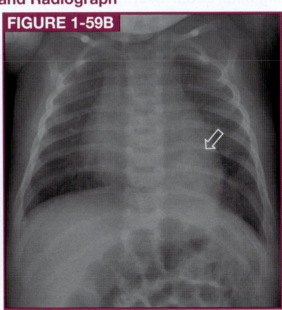

FIGURE 1-59B

This fetal MRI was obtained in a different patient with pulmonary sequestration. It demonstrates a T2 hyperintense mass in the left lower lobe (open arrows), with an anomalous vessel from the descending thoracic aorta extending to the lesion (arrow).

The postnatal frontal radiograph shows a vague retrocardiac opacity (open arrow), which correlates with the prenatal findings.

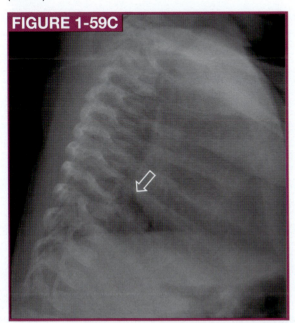

FIGURE 1-59C

The lateral postnatal radiograph confirms the left lower-lobe lung lesion (open arrow).

Congenital Lobar Overinflation (CLO)

Imaging Findings

CLO is characterized by progressive enlargement and hyperinflation of a portion of the lung, usually a single pulmonary lobe. The lobe may initially be only mildly hyperexpanded, retaining fetal fluid with increased density vs. normal lung parenchyma. Over time, it will clear of fluid and continue to expand, become markedly enlarged and hyperlucent, and displace the normal intrathoracic structures.

Clinical Correlation

Neonates with CLO have varying degrees of respiratory compromise at birth, but progressive respiratory distress will ultimately require lobectomy. The disease can be fatal if left untreated.

Key Points

- Prenatal diagnosis of CLO is also increasing with frequent use of high-quality prenatal imaging.

- The etiology of CLO is an abnormal bronchus that allows air to inflate the affected lobe, but obstructs it from leaving in a ball-valve effect.

Serial Progression of CLO

FIGURE 1-60A

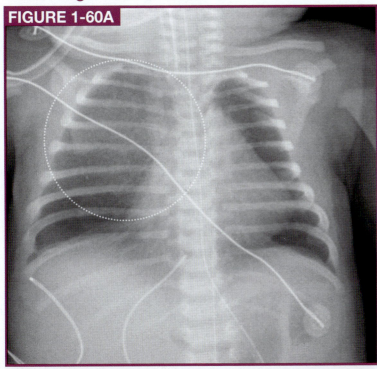

This chest radiograph obtained on the neonate's first day of life shows a mildly hyperinflated right upper lobe with hazy opacities compatible with retained fluid (dashed circle).

FIGURE 1-60B

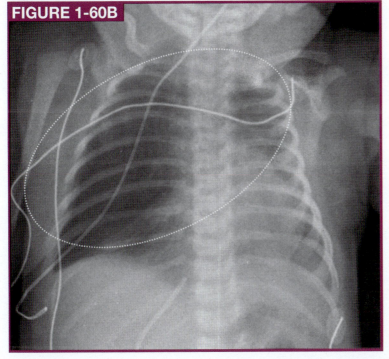

In an image obtained two days later, the right upper lobe has become severely hyperinflated (dashed oval), herniating into the left upper chest and causing leftward mediastinal shift. The involved lung is hyperlucent and the fetal lung fluid has cleared.

Bell-Shaped Chest

Imaging Findings

Bell-shaped chest is a nonspecific imaging finding in which flaring of the lower rib cage is secondary to disproportionate size between a smaller chest and a larger abdomen.

Clinical Correlation

If mild, a bell-shaped chest is indicative of generalized hypotonia from a variety of potential causes, including neurologic insult or neuromuscular pharmacologic blockade. A severe finding may suggest a more ominous diagnosis, such as skeletal dysplasia, trisomy 21, or bilateral pulmonary hypoplasia. If pulmonary hypoplasia is suspected – particularly if there is an associated air leak, such as pneumothorax or pneumomediastinum – ultrasound evaluation of kidneys for possible agenesis, dysplasia, or obstructive uropathy is imperative.

Key Points

- Bell-shaped chest is a nonspecific imaging finding.
- In the absence of chromosomal abnormality or skeletal dysplasia, renal ultrasound is recommended for patients with a severe deformity and air leak.

Bell-Shaped Chest With Pulmonary Hypoplasia

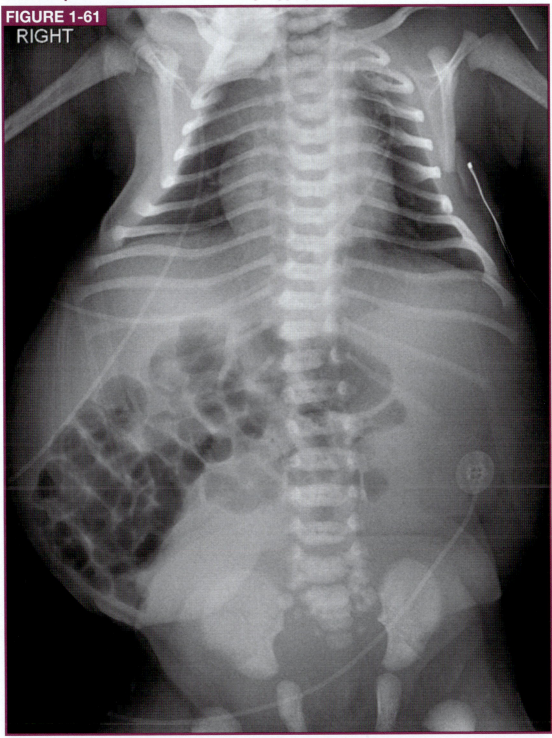

FIGURE 1-61
RIGHT

A bell-shaped chest is seen in this patient with prune belly syndrome. Weakness of the abdominal wall musculature and bilateral enlarged hydronephrotic kidneys have caused the flanks to bulge. The lungs and chest cavity are small due to associated pulmonary hypoplasia.

Esophageal Atresia/Tracheo-esophageal (TE) Fistula

Imaging Findings

Imaging can be used to support a clinical suspicion of esophageal atresia. Radiographs are frequently obtained to evaluate the position of an enteric tube that does not pass easily into the stomach. These images will show the tube coiled in the proximal esophagus. In cases of proximal esophageal atresia, air injected through the tube will demonstrate a gas-filled proximal esophageal pouch. The presence of distal bowel gas is an important indicator of TE fistula.

Clinical Correlation

Infants with esophageal atresia/TE fistula have difficulty feeding, during which they may cough, gag, or turn blue. Suspicion for the diagnosis increases when an enteric tube does not easily pass into the stomach.

Key Points

- There are many different subtypes of esophageal atresia. A combination of surgical, bronchoscopic, and imaging evaluation is often used to evaluate the esophageal and tracheal anatomy and to guide management.

- Esophageal atresia and TE fistula may occur in isolation, or may represent elements of VACTERL association. Evaluate radiographs carefully for evidence of cardiac disease, osseous anomalies, and distal bowel obstruction that may serve as clues to additional anatomic abnormalities.

Esophageal Atresia With TE Fistula

These radiographs show two patients with esophageal atresia. In both images, the presence of distal bowel gas indicates a TE fistula.

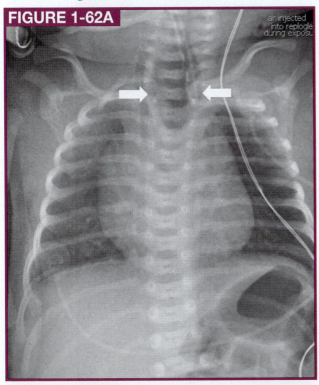

A dilated, gas-filled proximal esophageal pouch is present (arrows).

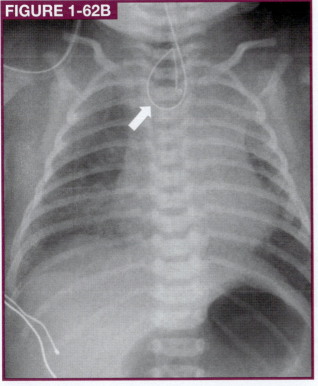

An enteric tube is coiled in the patient's proximal esophageal pouch (arrow).

Esophageal Atresia Without TE Fistula

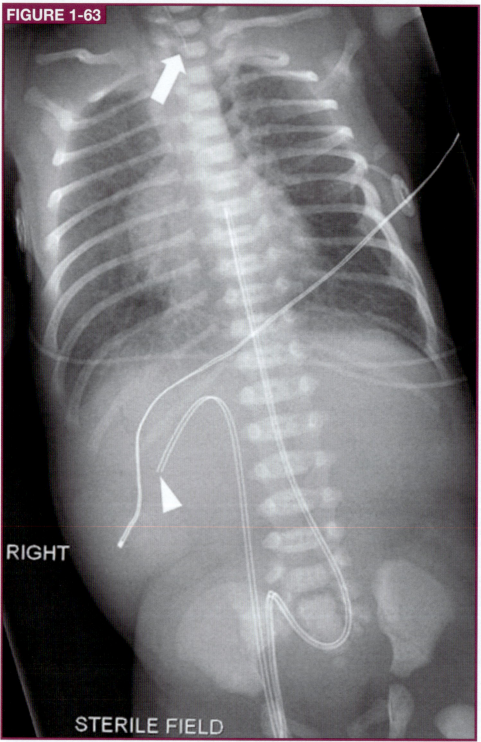

FIGURE 1-63

In this patient with esophageal atresia, an enteric tube cannot be passed beyond the proximal esophagus (arrow). The absence of bowel gas indicates that no TE fistula is present. A malpositioned umbilical venous catheter tip is noted over the liver (arrowhead).

Chylothorax

Imaging Findings

Chylothorax appears as pleural effusion, which is difficult to differentiate from other types of pleural fluid based on radiographic appearance alone. Diffuse interstitial densities in conjunction with a normal-sized heart may indicate lymphangiectasia, a common associated abnormality. The possibility of thoracic duct injury must be considered if surgical changes are present.

Clinical Correlation

Aspiration of pleural fluid in patients with chylothorax yields a milky lymphatic substance that contains fat microglobulins. Chylothorax can be seen in a variety of conditions, including congenital lymphangiectasia, lymphangiomatosis, Turner syndrome, Noonan syndrome, or after thoracic duct injury from surgery.

Key Points

- Serial radiographs may be obtained to monitor volume of the pleural fluid and evaluate efficacy of treatment.

Chylothorax With Lymphangiectasia

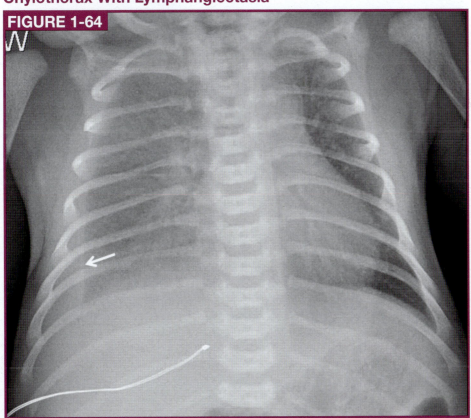

FIGURE 1-64

A right-sided pleural effusion (arrow) and diffuse interstitial densities are present in this patient with chylothorax due to lymphangiectasia.

Thoracic Neoplasm

Imaging Findings

Thoracic neoplasms are volume-positive processes that appear as masses on adjacent structures. Mediastinal deviation into the contralateral chest is common. Pleural effusion and osseous abnormalities, such as splaying of the ribs or focal erosions, may also be present.

Clinical Correlation

Although rare in neonates, thoracic neoplasms are cause for concern due to associated respiratory compromise and possible malignancy. Pathology ranges from benign vascular neoplasms to aggressive tumors. Surgical resection or biopsy is almost always required for diagnosis.

Key Points

- Subtle findings, such as calcifications, could be a clue to diagnosis. Stippled or coarse calcifications may be seen in cases of neuroblastoma or teratoma.

Thoracic Neoplasm Diagnosed as Teratoma

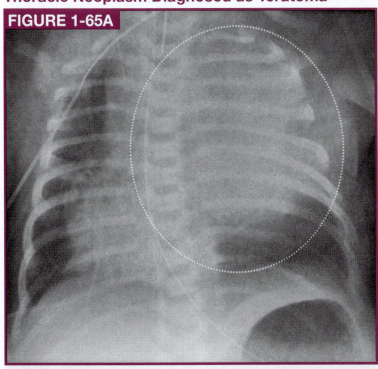

A large left-upper chest mass (dashed oval) causes rightward mediastinal deviation in this neonate.

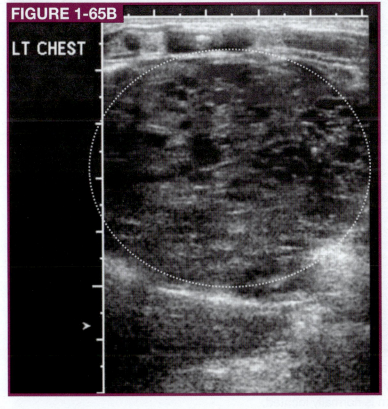

Ultrasound shows a heterogeneous solid lesion (dashed oval), with pathology ultimately revealing a teratoma.

Thoracic Neoplasm Diagnosed as Hemangioendothelioma

FIGURE 1-66

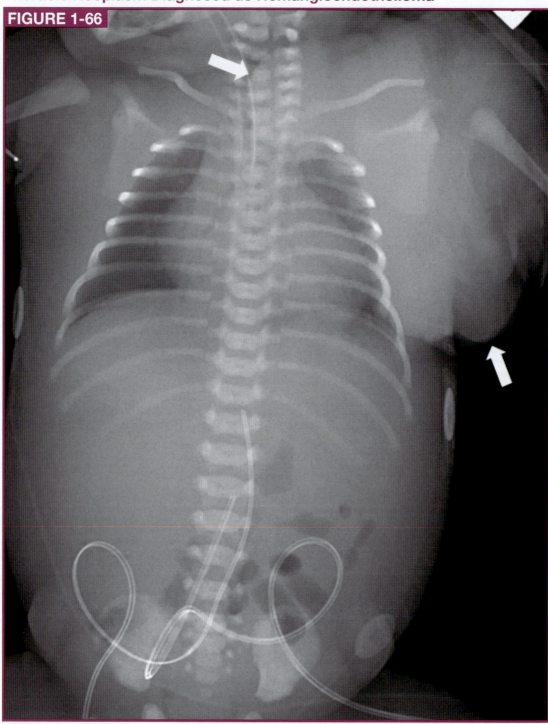

This patient was born with a large, superficial left upper-chest wall and axillary mass (arrows), which was ultimately diagnosed as a hemangioendothelioma. Because the tumor is extrathoracic, the mediastinum is normally located.

Chapter 2 The Neonatal Abdomen

TECHNIQUE

As with the chest, it is important to evaluate the adequacy of x-ray penetration when reading abdominal radiographs. Osseous structures and bowel gas will be visible on the study when appropriate technique is used. Often, organ outlines and peritoneal fat are also easily seen.

Adequate Penetration

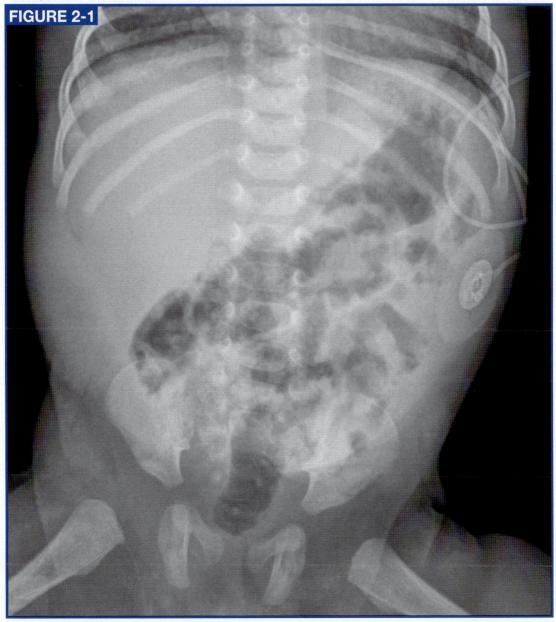

FIGURE 2-1

Adequate penetration allows visualization of osseous structures and bowel gas in this newborn's abdomen.

POSITIONING

The patient's positioning is also important when obtaining abdominal radiographs. The surface of the abdomen can significantly deviate from midline if the patient is rotated toward the right or the left. Therefore, a true anteroposterior view is critical to the evaluation of anterior structures.

Most abdominal radiographs are obtained with the patient in supine position while the x-ray beam passes from anterior to posterior. Other views can capitalize on the properties of gravity to demonstrate the position of gas in the abdomen. These include decubitus views, in which the patient's left or right side is positioned on the bed or table with the contralateral side directed toward the ceiling; and cross-table lateral views, in which the patient lies supine and the x-ray beam passes from right to left.

Supine, Decubitus, and Cross-Table Lateral Positioning

Pneumoperitoneum is demonstrated on three different views of the abdomen.

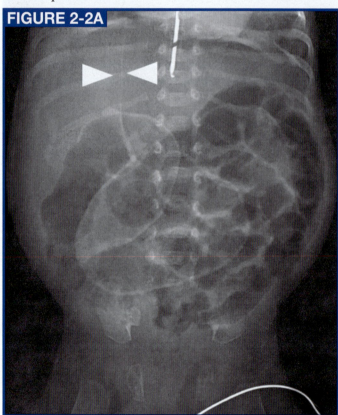

FIGURE 2-2A

Large-volume pneumperitoneum is subtly present on this supine frontal view. The falciform ligament is visible (arrowheads) and there is generalized lucency in the upper abdomen, indicating free gas.

FIGURE 2-2B

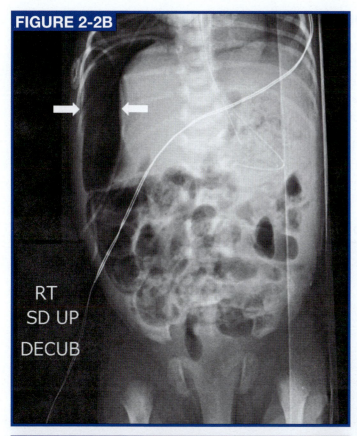

A left-lateral decubitus view of the abdomen more clearly shows pneumoperitoneum layering over the liver (arrows).

FIGURE 2-2C

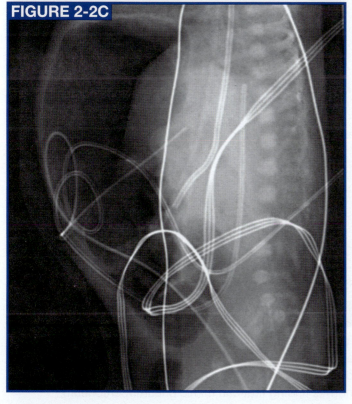

The cross-table lateral view shows free gas that has risen to the nondependent portion of the abdomen.

NORMAL ABDOMINAL RADIOGRAPH

Bowel gas pattern is a critical item to evaluate on an abdominal radiograph. Normal position of the stomach and proximal bowel loops are in the left upper quadrant, the liver in the right upper quadrant, and the cecum in the right lower quadrant. Any variation could indicate a situs abnormality or intestinal malrotation, and should be further investigated with fluoroscopic examination or ultrasound.

In the immediate postnatal period, bowel gas may be seen only in the stomach and proximal small intestine. It should be seen in the distal colon and rectum by 24 hours, and is often present at six to eight hours of life.

Normal Radiograph With No Distal Bowel Gas

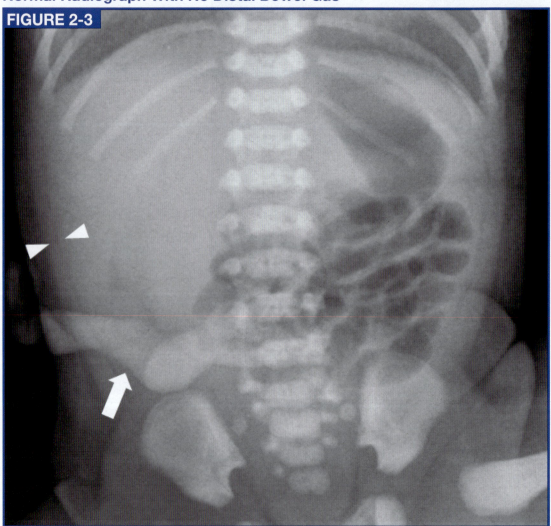

FIGURE 2-3

This supine anteroposterior view of the abdomen, obtained in the infant's first few hours of life, shows gas within the stomach and proximal bowel loops, but not in the distal bowel. A long umbilical stump is still attached (arrow). A well-defined peritoneal fat stripe is also clearly visualized (arrowheads), which is a normal finding that can mimic pneumoperitoneum.

Normal Bowel Gas Pattern

Normal bowel loops tend to collapse on each other and appear as multiple small, superimposed, polygonal shapes. Bowel gas should be scattered throughout the abdomen.

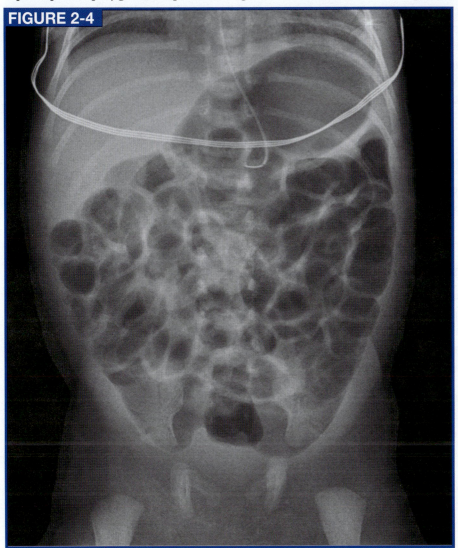

FIGURE 2-4

This neonate's bowel is gas-filled but not dilated, with collapsed loops superimposed on one another. The enteric tube is in satisfactory position, with the tip terminating over the gastric body.

Consider the following if bowel obstruction is suspected: In general, the diameter of any single loop of bowel should never be larger than the transverse dimension of a lumbar spine vertebral body, and dilated bowel loops may display a tubular morphology. The presence of intraluminal gas-fluid levels is not normal in the neonatal period and could indicate bowel obstruction. Absence of bowel gas in the distal colon and rectum can support a diagnosis of bowel obstruction, but is nonspecific.

It is important to consider that bowel loops tend to be featureless in the neonatal period. Therefore, differentiation between the small and large bowel can be difficult.

LINES AND TUBES

Radiographs are often obtained to evaluate or confirm the position of supportive lines and tubes. The tip of the line or tube is often described as terminating "over" a structure of interest, as the exact position cannot be determined by a single two-dimensional image. Generally, if an enteric tube tip terminates "over" the stomach, it likely terminates in the stomach. However, rare instances of hollow viscus or vascular perforation do occur, particularly in the setting of difficult placement or extreme prematurity. Exercise caution if an unusual clinical course or imaging features are present. Additional views obtained in an orthogonal plane to the initial study can help to further evaluate positioning of support devices.

Umbilical Catheters

Umbilical catheters provide vascular access in the immediate postnatal period. Adjustments are often required after placement to achieve optimal positioning and avoid associated complications.

Umbilical Venous Catheters (UVCs)

UVCs should extend through the umbilical vein at the umbilicus, course along the anterior midline or right paramedian abdomen, and pass through the liver posteriorly through the left portal vein and ductus venosus into the inferior vena cava. The normal position of the catheter tip is at the junction of the inferior vena cava and the right atrium, also known as the inferior cavoatrial junction.

UVCs pass several venous confluences on the way to the inferior vena cava. Therefore, they can sometimes deviate into one of these structures, most commonly into one of the branches of the portal vein. They can also become looped or kinked within the vascular structures. If a catheter is placed too proximally, the tip will miss its targeted central location. Alternatively, a catheter that is advanced too far may extend through a patent foramen ovale or atrial septal defect into the left atrium, cross the tricuspid valve into the right ventricle, or continue through the right atrium into the superior vena cava.

Normal Course of UVC

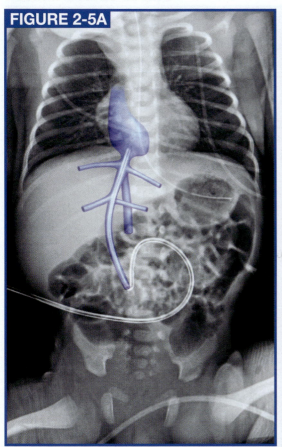

Normal course of a UVC on a frontal radiograph.

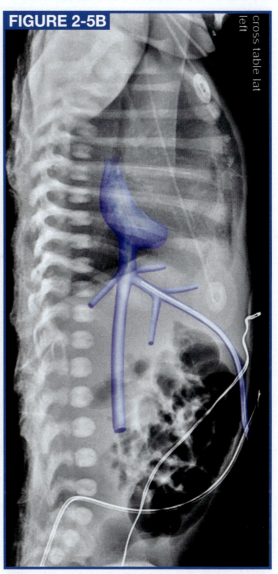

Normal course of a UVC on a lateral radiograph.

UVC Deviation Into the Portal Vein

FIGURE 2-6

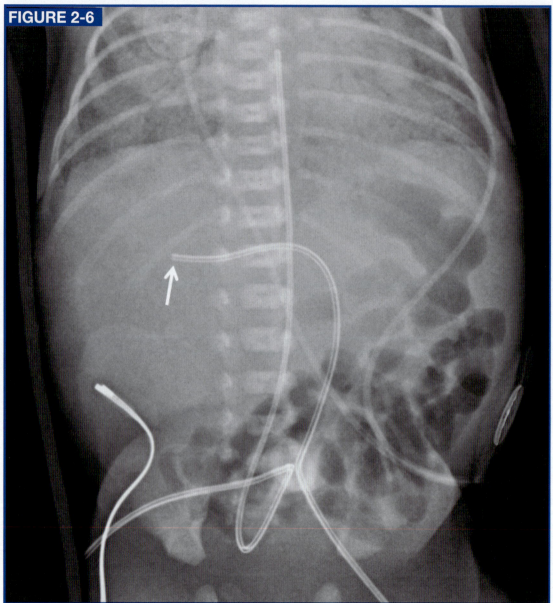

This UVC deviates to the right, likely within the right branch of the portal vein (arrow). Malpositioning of the catheter into the portal vein may cause abscess, thrombosis, or hemorrhage.

UVC Deviation Into the Splenic Vein

FIGURE 2-7

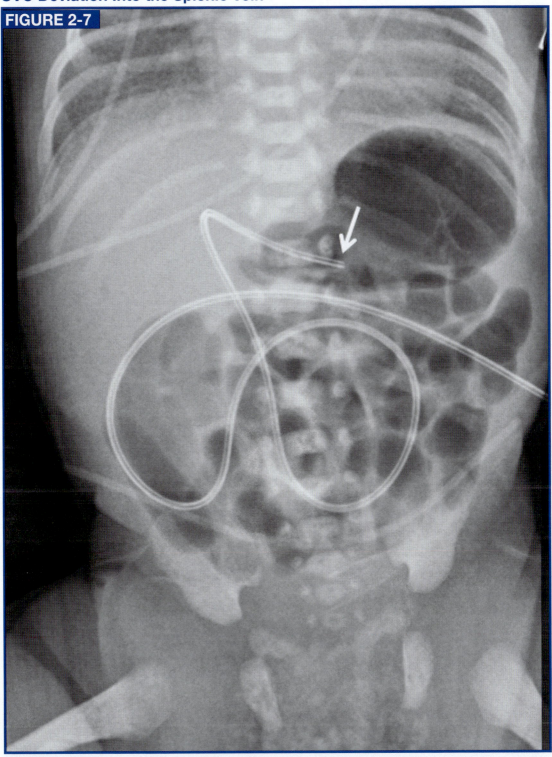

This malpositioned catheter likely extends into the splenic vein (arrow).

UVC Deviation Into the Left Atrium

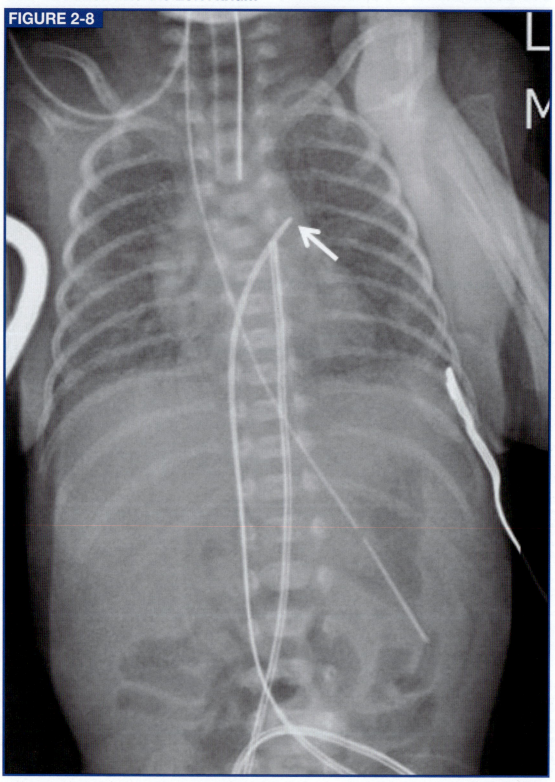

FIGURE 2-8

This UVC extends too far superiorly, and has likely passed through a patent foramen ovale into the left atrium, possibly into a pulmonary vein (arrow).

UVC Deviation Into the Superior Vena Cava

FIGURE 2-9

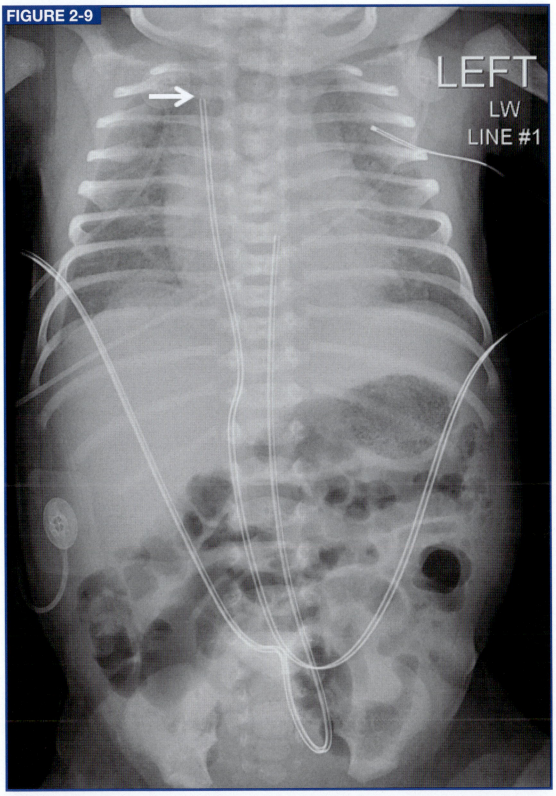

This UVC also extends too far superiorly. Its tip overlies the superior vena cava (arrow).

UVC Coiled Over the Liver

FIGURE 2-10

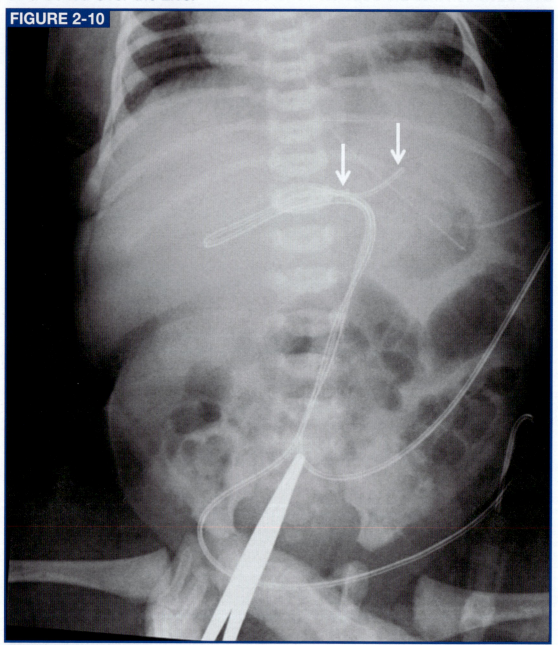

Placement of two UVCs was attempted in this patient. Both catheters are coiled over the liver (arrows).

Low Anterior UVC Positioning

This patient's UVC has taken an unusual course.

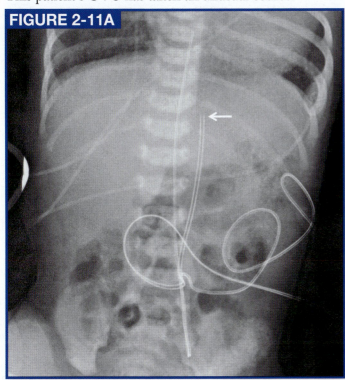

FIGURE 2-11A

The frontal view shows that the tip is positioned too low at the level of the T11-T12 interspace (arrow).

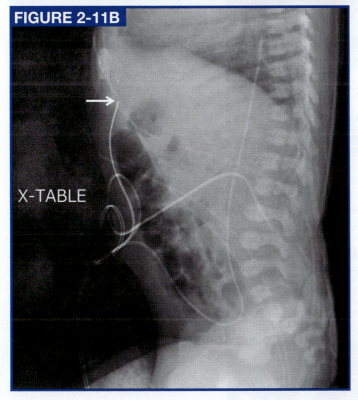

FIGURE 2-11B

The lateral view shows that the catheter is too anterior (arrow). It was promptly removed following review.

Umbilical Artery Catheters (UACs)

UACs are placed into one of the paired umbilical arteries. The catheter should initially course inferiorly and posteriorly, enter into the right or left iliac artery, then ascend into the abdominal aorta and, possibly, the thoracic aorta. Proper positioning decreases the risk of iatrogenic vascular injury and thromboembolic phenomenon.

There are two acceptable UAC positions. The "high" position, with the tip between the level of the T6 and T10 vertebral bodies, avoids the major branches of the thoracic aorta, specifically the subclavian artery. The "low" position, with the tip between the level of the L3 and L5 vertebral bodies, avoids the major branches of the abdominal aorta that supply the kidneys and intestines.

Normal High Position of UAC

One helpful indicator of an umbilical catheter that is arterial rather than venous is its initial inferior course as it approaches the iliac artery prior to coursing superiorly into the aorta. The tip of this infant's catheter is in the normal high position.

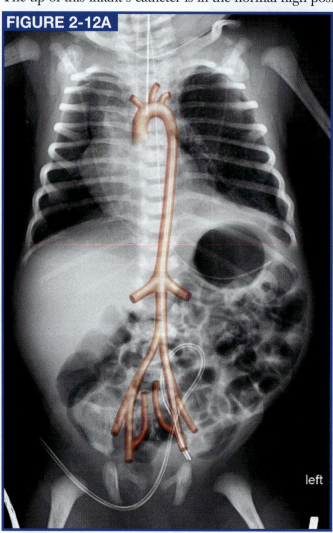

Normal course of a UAC on a frontal radiograph.

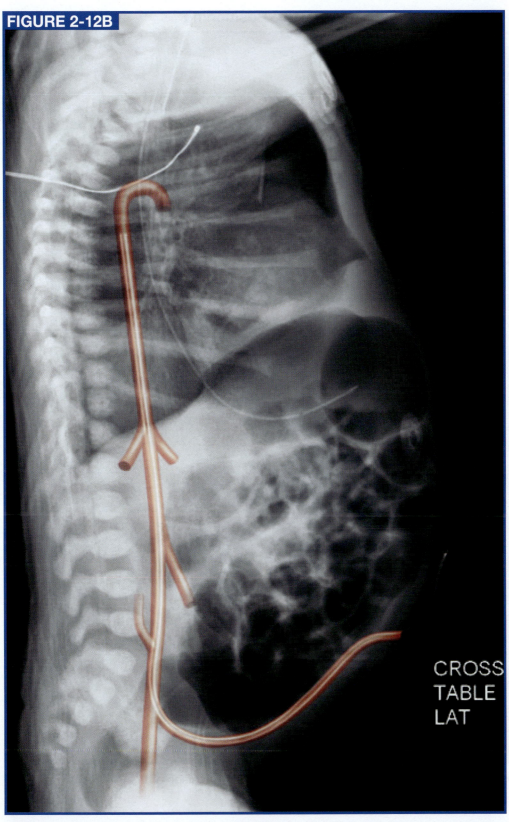

Normal course of a UAC on a lateral radiograph.

Cross-Table Lateral View of High UAC Positioning

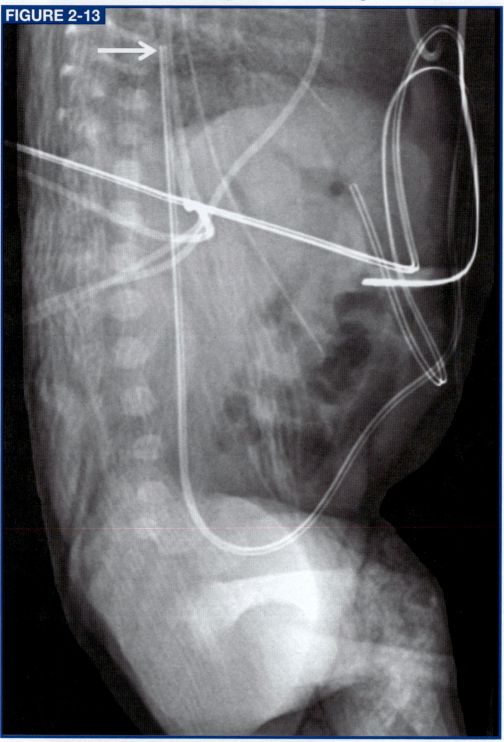

FIGURE 2-13

This cross-table lateral view shows the expected posterior position of the UAC as it courses superiorly through the aorta (arrow).

Normal Low Position of UAC

FIGURE 2-14

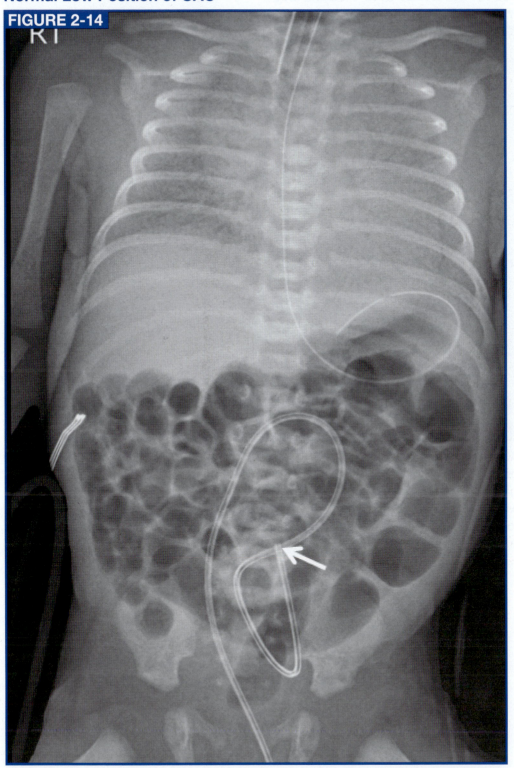

This image shows a UAC in a normal low position, with the tip at the level of the L4 vertebral body (arrow).

Correct vs. Incorrect UAC Positioning

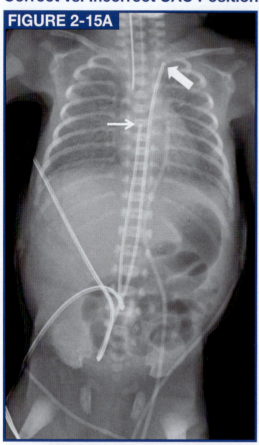

FIGURE 2-15A

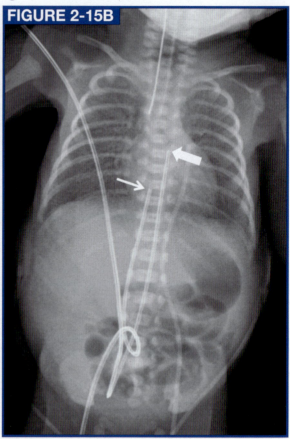

FIGURE 2-15B

The UAC (thick arrow) extends too far superiorly on the initial image, likely near the origin of the left common carotid or subclavian artery. The UVC (thin arrow) is also too high, projecting over the superior right atrium.

After retraction, the UAC (thick arrow) is in appropriate position, with the tip at the level of the T6 vertebral body. The UVC (thin arrow) now projects slightly above the inferior cavoatrial junction.

Looped UAC

FIGURE 2-16

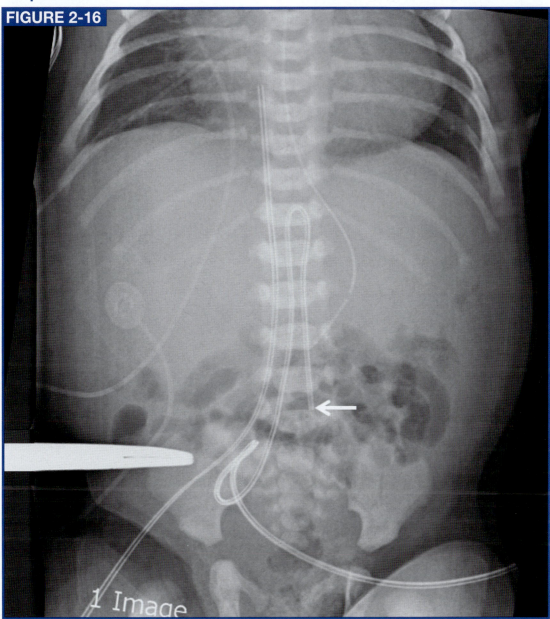

The UAC in this image is looped in the abdominal aorta and needs to be removed (arrow).

UAC Over Right Iliac Artery

FIGURE 2-17

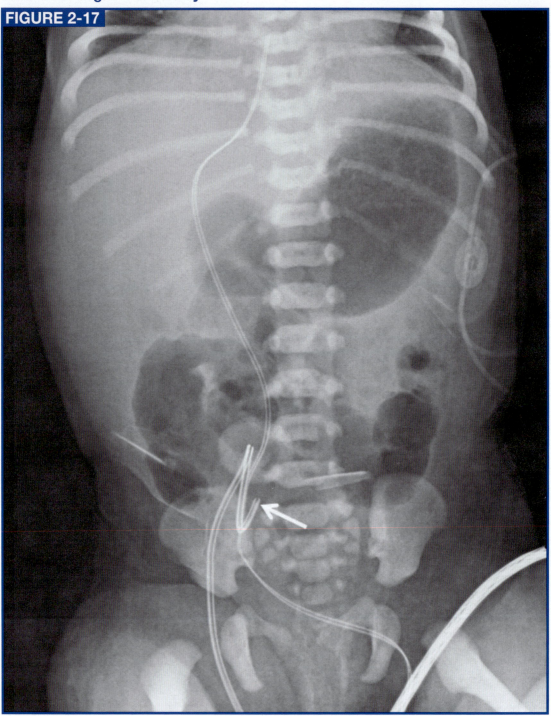

This UAC is malpositioned, with the tip overlying the right iliac artery (arrow).

Peripherally Inserted Central Catheters (PICCs)

When umbilical catheters cannot be used, PICCs are commonly placed to maintain vascular access, administer medications, and provide parenteral nutrition. If a lower extremity is the site of access, the PICC should course superiorly into the iliac veins and inferior vena cava. The PICC tip should ideally terminate at the junction of the right atrium and inferior vena cava.

Lower Extremity PICC Positioning

Lower extremity PICCs are typically inserted in the saphenous vein and pass through the common femoral and iliac veins into the inferior vena cava. The tip should ideally terminate in the inferior vena cava at its junction with the right atrium (the inferior cavoatrial junction).

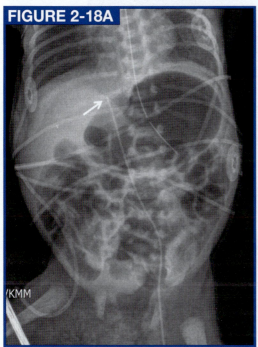

Frontal radiograph of the abdomen showing a left lower-extremity PICC with the tip near the inferior cavoatrial junction (arrow).

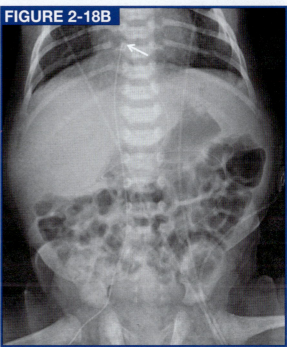

In a different baby, a right lower-extremity PICC tip overlies the inferior right atrium just above the inferior cavoatrial junction (arrow).

PICC Deviation Into the Left Atrium

FIGURE 2-19

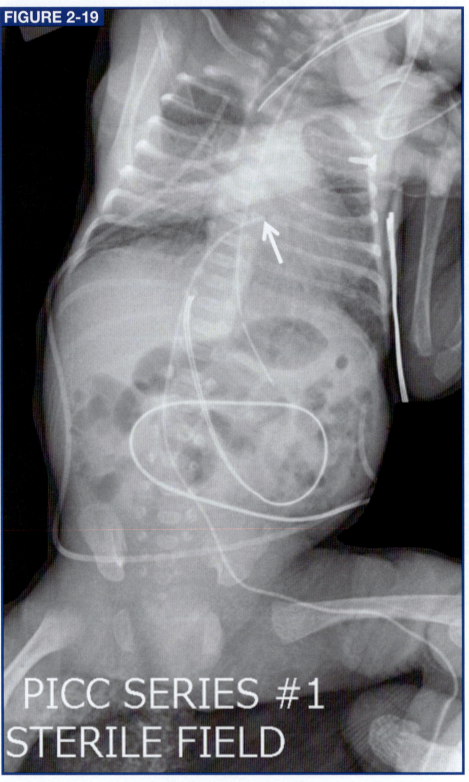

This left lower-extremity PICC has passed into the right atrium, crossing the patent foramen ovale into the left atrium (arrow). Repositioning is necessary.

PICC Deviation Into a Lumbar Vein

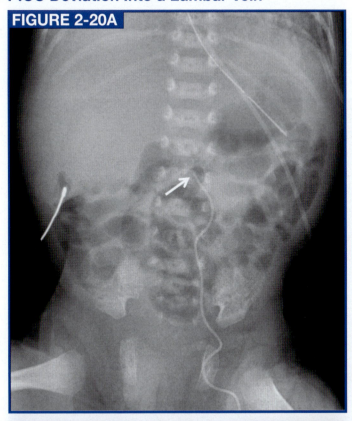

FIGURE 2-20A

The left lower-extremity PICC in this 25-week-premature infant has an unusual serpentine appearance (arrow) and does not cross the midline along the expected course of the inferior vena cava.

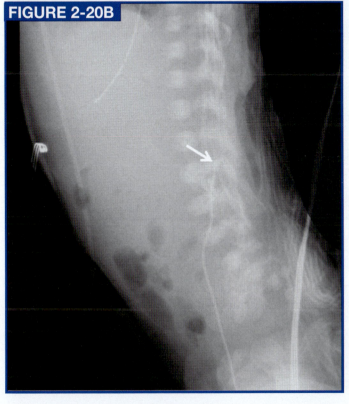

FIGURE 2-20B

On the cross-table lateral view, the tip projects posteriorly over the spine, where it has entered a lumbar vein (arrow).

Enteric Tubes

Enteric tubes are used to administer nutritional support or provide suction of enteric contents.

Enteric Tube Positioning for Nutritional Support

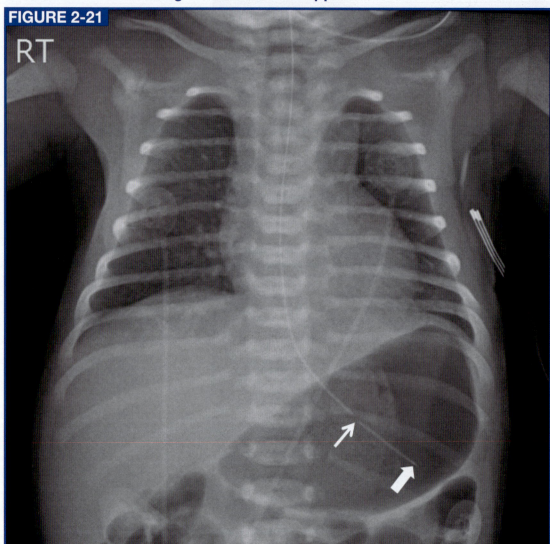

FIGURE 2-21

The side port and tip of an enteric tube used for nutritional support should project over the stomach or small bowel. In this image, the side port (thin arrow) and tip (thick arrow) of the enteric tube project over the gastric body. A tube that is too proximal increases the risk of reflux and aspiration when feeding material is administered. Ensure that the tube follows the expected course of the esophagus. Endobronchial placement is rare, but can result in serious illness or death.

Enteric tubes used for suctioning should also have the side port and tip over the stomach. Chronic suction on esophageal mucosa can cause perforation or permanent damage.

Enteric Tube Positioning With Gastric Perforation

FIGURE 2-22A

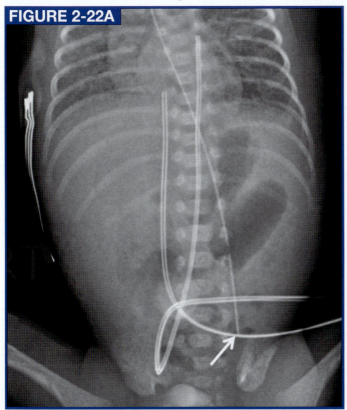

In this extremely low birth weight (ELBW) infant, an enteric tube was advanced too far. The tip is in the left lower quadrant, inferior to the gastric bubble (arrow). Visualization of the falciform ligament is a very subtle finding of free peritoneal gas.

FIGURE 2-22B

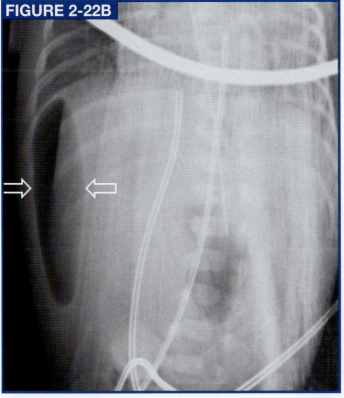

A follow-up left-lateral decubitus view of the abdomen more clearly shows pneumoperitoneum, confirming gastric perforation.

Incorrectly Sized Enteric Tube

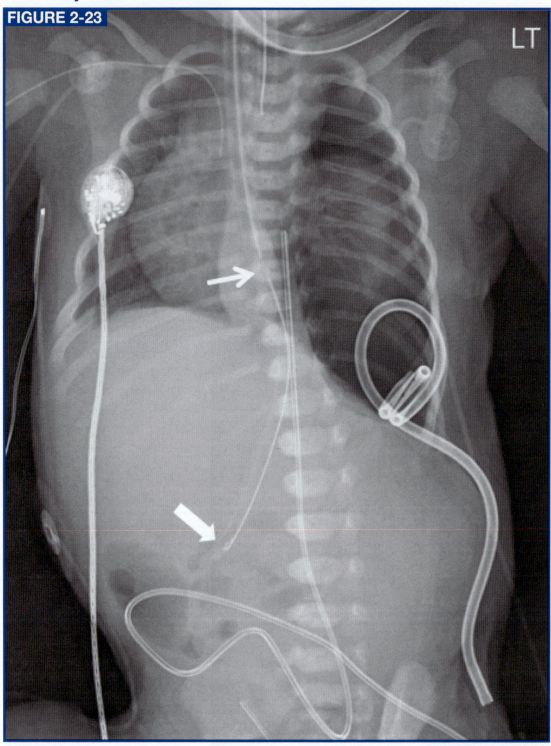

FIGURE 2-23

It is important to choose the correct size of enteric tube for the neonate. This image shows an infant with a congenital diaphragmatic hernia (CDH) repair. The side port of the enteric tube overlies the distal thoracic esophagus (thin arrow), but the tip is well within the stomach (thick arrow). It should be replaced with a smaller tube.

THE PERIPHERY: BONES AND SOFT TISSUES

As with the chest, careful evaluation of the non-target structures — bones, subcutaneous tissues, diaphragm, and lower lungs — is an important step in interpreting abdominal radiographs. Care should be taken to look for vertebral anomalies, fractures, and findings of metabolic disease.

Congenital Osseous Abnormalities Visible on Abdominal Radiograph

FIGURE 2-24

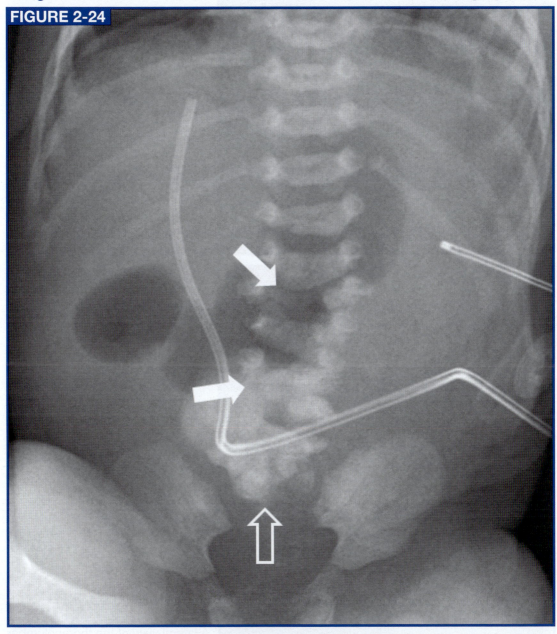

Multiple vertebral anomalies (solid arrows) and a hypoplastic sacrum (open arrow) are present in this neonate. These types of osseous abnormalities should raise suspicion for associated anatomic anomalies in other organ systems.

Caudal Regression Syndrome Visible on Abdominal Radiograph

Images of an infant with caudal regression syndrome. Patients with this disease may have associated motor-sensory and genitourinary abnormalities of varying degrees.

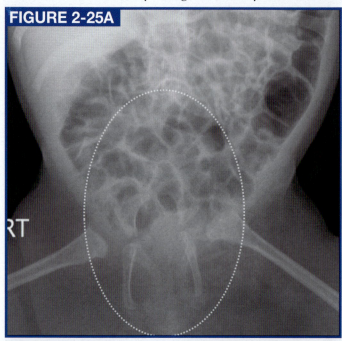

FIGURE 2-25A

A frontal view of the abdomen reveals absent lumbar vertebral bodies, absent sacrum, and a small pelvis (dashed oval).

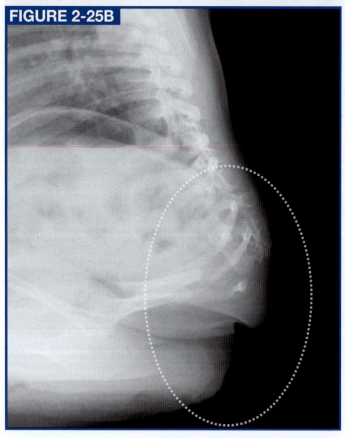

FIGURE 2-25B

A lateral view of the thoracolumbar spine also shows truncation of the lumbar spine with an absent sacrum (dashed oval).

Chondrodysplasia Punctata Visible on Abdominal Radiograph

FIGURE 2-26

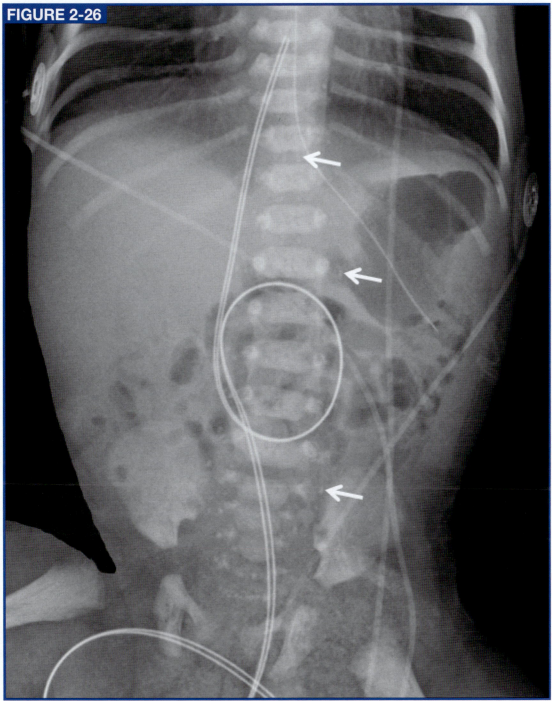

Here, subtle stippled calcifications associated with the osseous structures (arrows) are indicative of chondrodysplasia punctata, which is a spectrum of skeletal dysplasias that include lethal forms.

Fetal Hydrops Visible on Abdominal Radiograph

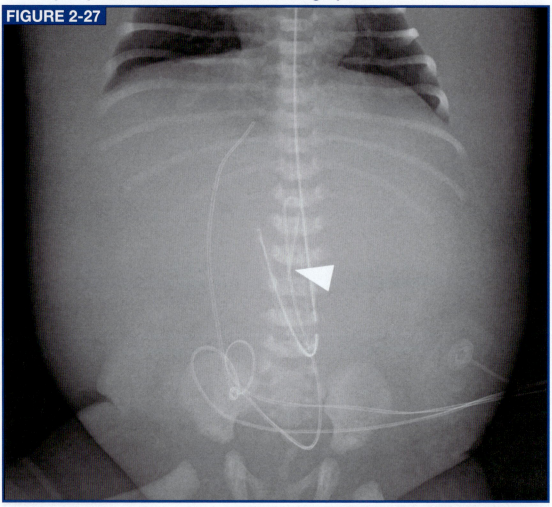

FIGURE 2-27

This radiograph was ordered to evaluate positioning of a neonate's support lines and tubes. It shows an absent bowel gas pattern and severe body wall edema, which are compatible with a clinical history of fetal hydrops. Note that the UAC is looped over the abdominal aorta (arrowhead) and needs to be removed or repositioned.

Inguinal Hernia Visible on Abdominal Radiograph

FIGURE 2-28

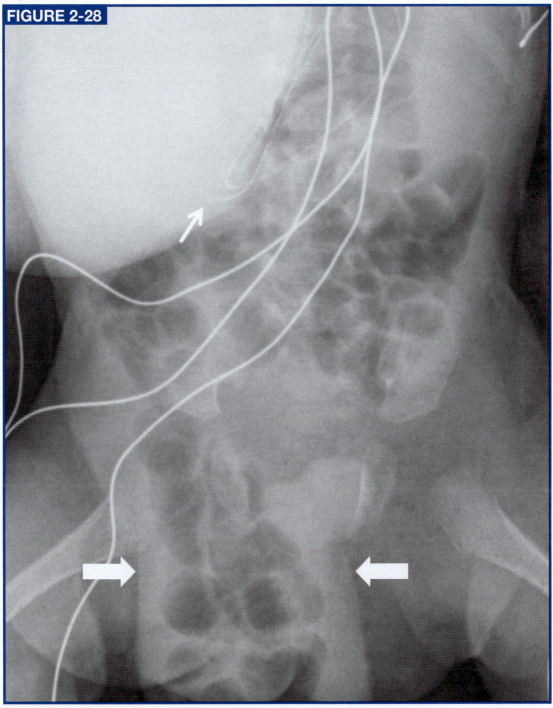

This newborn infant with a giant omphalocele has a large, right-sided, bowel-containing inguinal hernia on radiographic examination (thick arrows). The enteric tube is coiled over the stomach in the upper abdomen (thin arrow).

Femur Fracture Visible on Abdominal Radiograph

FIGURE 2-29

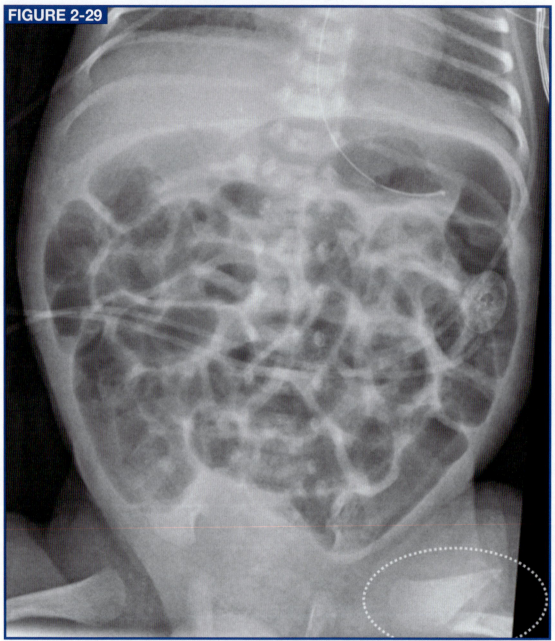

A left femur fracture is demonstrated at the inferior margin of this abdominal radiograph (dashed oval).

PATHOLOGY

Pneumoperitoneum

Imaging Findings

Pneumoperitoneum may manifest as a generalized lucency over the upper abdomen. Intraperitoneal gas may outline the falciform ligament, which is referred to as the "football sign" and should never appear on a normal abdominal radiograph. The presence of gas on the intraluminal and extraluminal sides of the bowel wall, called the "Rigler sign" or "double wall sign," is also abnormal. Small triangles of free gas can sometimes be seen outside the bowel wall. Free intraperitoneal gas that outlines the entire inferior margin of the diaphragm is referred to as the "continuous diaphragm sign." These radiographic signs of pneumoperitoneum are rarely all present. Commonly, only one or two are demonstrated. Occasionally, pneumoperitoneum is entirely nonvisible on a supine view.

Clinical Correlation

Neonates with unexpected pneumoperitoneum require urgent treatment to prevent abdominal compartment syndrome and to treat the underlying cause. The surgical team should be consulted to aid in evaluation and management.

Key Points

- Discovery of pneumoperitoneum can significantly alter the treatment of an ill neonate. However, it can be very challenging to identify free gas, especially on a supine image. Obtaining a left-lateral decubitus or cross-table lateral view will help to confirm the diagnosis.

- Patients with necrotizing enterocolitis, toxic megacolon, or iatrogenic injury should be closely scrutinized for evidence of pneumoperitoneum.

Pneumoperitoneum With Football and Rigler Signs

This ELBW infant developed pneumoperitoneum in association with spontaneous bowel perforation.

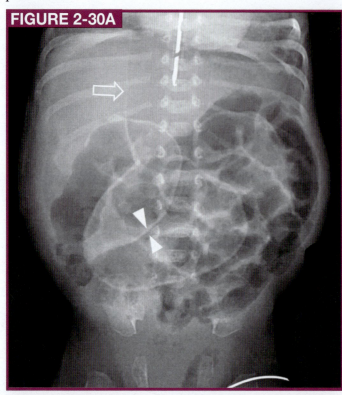

The falciform ligament is clearly visualized over the liver, compatible with the football sign (open arrow). The Rigler sign is also present (arrowheads)

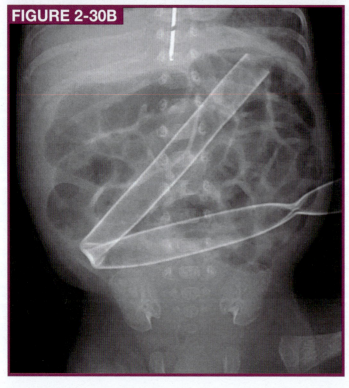

The pneumoperitoneum is nearly completely resolved after placement of a surgical drain. Note that the enteric tube, with side holes projecting over the distal thoracic esophagus, should be advanced further into the stomach.

Pneumoperitoneum With Continuous Diaphragm and Rigler Signs

FIGURE 2-31

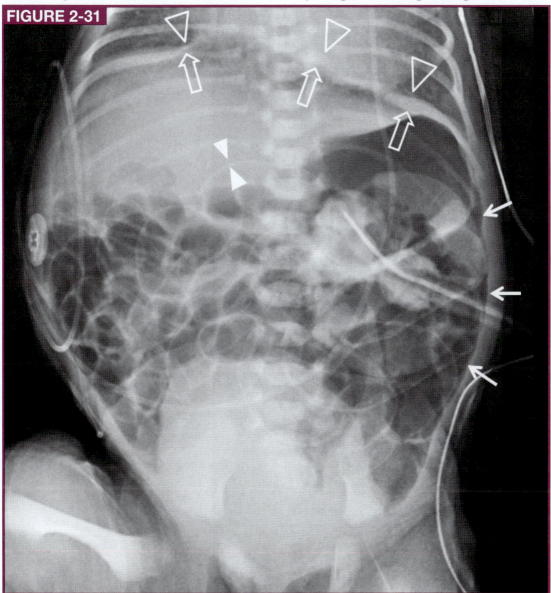

Another infant with large-volume pneumoperitoneum shows a continuous diaphragm sign (open arrowheads superiorly and open arrows inferiorly), Rigler sign (arrowheads), and small, extraluminal lucent triangles of gas (arrows).

Supine vs. Left-Lateral Decubitus Pneumoperitoneum Views

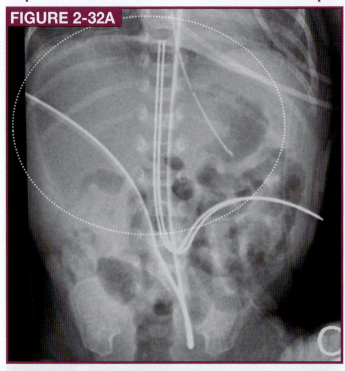

A frontal abdominal radiograph in a neonate with pneumoperitoneum demonstrates abnormal lucency overlying the upper abdomen (dashed oval).

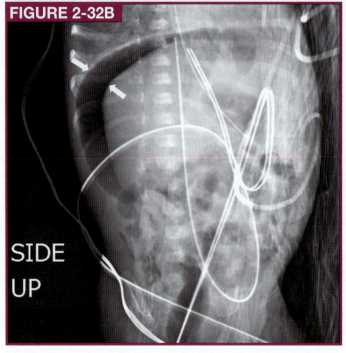

Extraluminal gas clearly outlines the liver on the left-lateral decubitus view (arrows).

Subtle Findings of Pneumoperitoneum

More subtle findings of pneumoperitoneum are present in this premature infant.

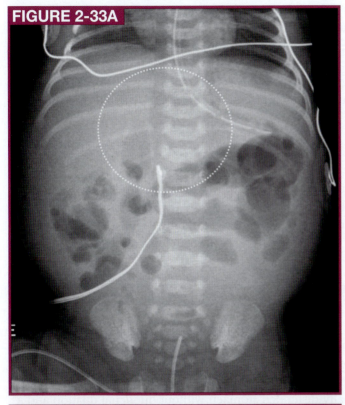

FIGURE 2-33A

Vague lucencies overlie the liver on the frontal view (dashed circle).

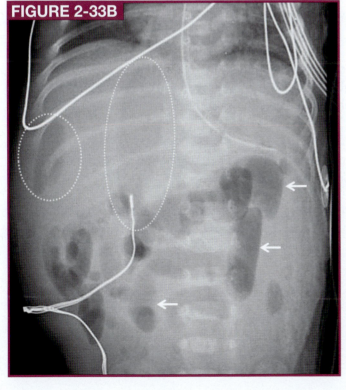

FIGURE 2-33B

Two abnormal loculated gas collections are evident on the left-lateral decubitus view (dashed ovals). There is no bowel normally overlying the liver in this location to explain these lucencies. Several gas-fluid levels in the bowel are present, denoting necrotizing enterocolitis (arrows).

Bowel Obstruction

Numerous anatomic and functional causes of gastrointestinal obstruction are possible in the perinatal period. Patients may present with emesis, which may be bilious or nonbilious, depending on the location of the obstruction relative to the site of biliary drainage in the duodenum. Other indicators include delayed passage of meconium, abdominal distension, and feeding intolerance. Intestinal perforation is a rare but potentially serious complication. Definitive treatment varies according to the cause of obstruction. Nearly all cases require surgical consultation to aid in evaluation and management. Most require some type of operative intervention.

Proximal Bowel Obstruction

Common causes of proximal gastrointestinal obstruction in neonates include gastric outlet obstruction due to pyloric stenosis; duodenal obstruction due to duodenal atresia, duodenal stenosis, duodenal web, annular pancreas, or malrotation with midgut volvulus; and jejunal atresia. Radiographs can narrow the differential diagnosis and guide next steps.

Hypertrophic Pyloric Stenosis (HPS)

Imaging Findings

Targeted abdominal ultrasound of the pyloric region is the test of choice for HPS. Findings include abnormal thickening and elongation of the pyloric wall musculature and failure of gastric contents to pass through the pyloric channel. If an abdominal radiograph is obtained, findings typically include an abnormally distended stomach without duodenal dilation and a small amount of gas within nondilated loops of distal bowel.

Clinical Correlation

HPS is an idiopathic condition that causes gastric outlet obstruction due to abnormal thickening of the pyloric wall musculature. Patients present with forceful nonbilious vomiting. Evidence of dehydration and electrolyte imbalance may also be seen.

Key Points

- HPS typically presents in infants between three and 12 weeks of age. HPS outside of this range is much less likely, but atypical cases do occur.

- A surgical incision along the length of the pyloric wall muscle is required to relieve the gastric outlet obstruction.

HPS on Radiograph and Ultrasound

Imaging performed on an infant with projectile nonbilious vomiting.

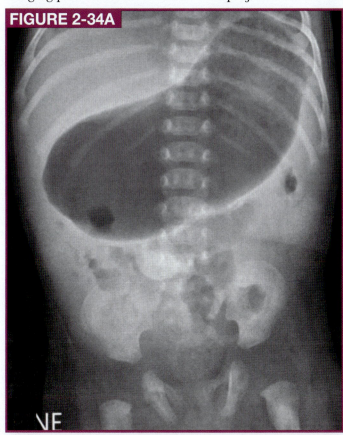

FIGURE 2-34A

An abdominal radiograph shows marked gaseous distension of the stomach with scattered gas in nondilated distal bowel loops. The duodenum is not dilated.

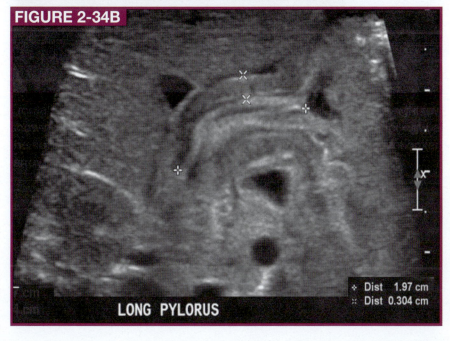

FIGURE 2-34B

An ultrasound of the same patient reveals abnormal thickening ("x" markers) and elongation ("+" markers) of the pyloric muscle, compatible with HPS.

Duodenal Atresia/Duodenal Stenosis

Imaging Findings

Patients with duodenal atresia will typically have an enlarged gastric bubble and proximal duodenum, creating a "double bubble" appearance on radiograph. Normally, the nondilated duodenum cannot be differentiated from other surrounding bowel loops. Complete obstruction of the duodenum prevents passage of gas into more distal bowel loops. These findings are diagnostic, and further imaging is not required. Radiographic evaluation for duodenal atresia is more difficult after gastric decompression with an enteric tube.

Duodenal stenosis has a similar appearance to duodenal atresia, except that some distal bowel gas is present due to incomplete obstruction.

Clinical Correlation

Duodenal atresia and stenosis may be diagnosed by prenatal imaging. Patients will have bilious or nonbilious emesis after birth, depending on which portion of the duodenum has the atretic/stenotic segment. If left untreated, dehydration, weight loss, and electrolyte imbalance may occur.

Key Points

- Although they can occur in isolation, duodenal atresia and stenosis are more highly associated with genetic aberrancies, including trisomy 21, than are other causes of bowel obstruction. Dysmorphic findings of Down syndrome or other radiographic abnormalities, including presence of 11 paired ribs, flat acetabuluar angles, or evidence of congenital heart defect, can increase confidence in the diagnosis.

Duodenal Atresia With Double Bubble Sign

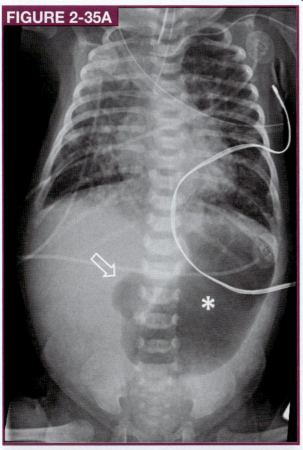

FIGURE 2-35A

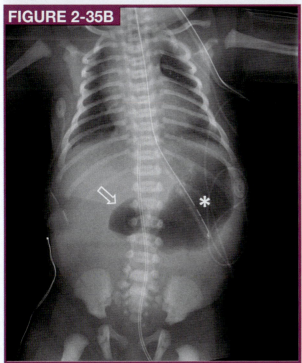

FIGURE 2-35B

A dilated gas-filled stomach (asterisks) and proximal duodenum, or double bubble sign (open arrows), is seen on radiographs of two different patients diagnosed with duodenal atresia.

Duodenal Stenosis with Double Bubble Sign

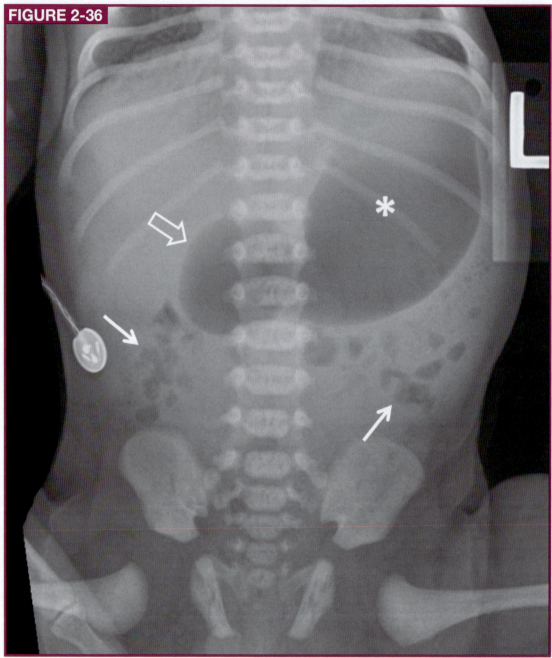

FIGURE 2-36

In addition to the dilated stomach (asterisk) and duodenum (open arrow), a small amount of distal bowel gas (arrows) is also seen on this radiograph of a patient with duodenal stenosis. A fluoroscopic upper GI examination should be performed to further evaluate the anatomy and to determine the location and severity of the obstruction.

Duodenal Web

Imaging Findings

Radiographic signs of duodenal web are similar to other types of duodenal obstruction and include distention of the stomach and a gas-filled, dilated proximal duodenum. Distal bowel gas is present because the obstruction is incomplete. A fluoroscopic upper GI study will provide further evaluation of the anatomy and determine the location and severity of the obstruction.

Clinical Correlation

Patients with duodenal web may present with feeding intolerance, poor weight gain, vomiting, or symptoms of gastroesophageal reflux.

Key Points

- A significantly dilated proximal duodenum is an important indicator of long-standing obstruction that helps distinguish duodenal web from other causes of acute bowel obstruction, such as midgut volvulus, which require emergent surgical intervention.

- The obstruction is caused by abnormal tissue that extends across the bowel lumen. Often, a pinhole opening permits small amounts of food or contrast to pass. The opening may decrease over time and worsen the obstruction.

Duodenal Web With Dilated Proximal Duodenum

Imaging in a patient with a duodenal web.

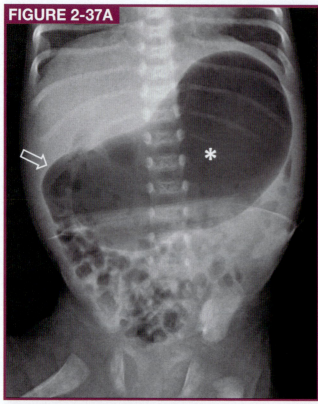

This abdominal radiograph shows marked gaseous distension of the stomach (asterisk) and proximal duodenum (open arrow).

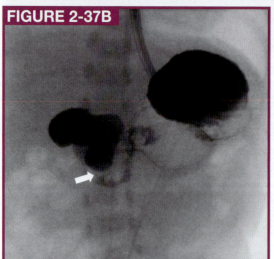

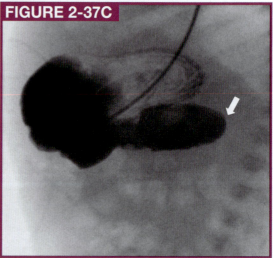

Frontal projection from a follow-up upper GI examination reveals a dilated proximal duodenum with an abrupt caliber change near the junction of the second and third duodenal segments (arrow). There is passage of only a small amount of contrast distally.

Lateral projection from the upper GI examination confirms the dilated proximal duodenum and associated partial obstruction (arrow).

Annular Pancreas

Imaging Findings

Radiographic manifestations of annular pancreas are similar to other forms of duodenal obstruction, with a double bubble present on a supine view. Distal bowel gas is present. fluoroscopic, CT, and MRI findings are more specific to the diagnosis.

Clinical Correlation

Similar to other forms of duodenal obstruction, patients may present with abdominal distension, feeding intolerance, and weight loss. Emesis is more commonly nonbilious than bilious.

Key Points

- Annular pancreas is the presence of abnormal pancreatic tissue surrounding the second portion of the duodenum due to abnormal embryologic formation of the pancreas. It can be complete or incomplete.

- The severity of duodenal narrowing and obstruction is linked to the age of the patient at presentation. Most are symptomatic and present in the neonatal period.

Example of Annular Pancreas on Fluoroscopy

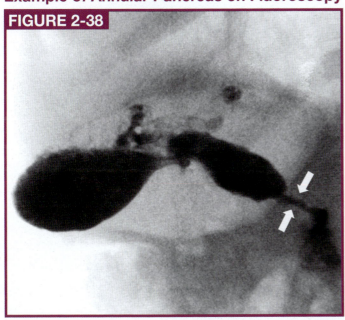

FIGURE 2-38

A lateral fluoroscopic image of an infant with emesis secondary to annular pancreas demonstrates marked narrowing of the second portion of the duodenum (arrows), with passage of a small amount of contrast material distally. A plain radiograph would show a distended stomach and proximal duodenum, similar to other types of duodenal obstruction.

Malrotation With Midgut Volvulus

Imaging Findings

Fluoroscopic images are essential to the diagnosis of intestinal malrotation with midgut volvulus. Abdominal radiographs are often nonspecific or appear normal, and are more helpful to evaluate for other causes of bilious emesis, including distal bowel obstruction.

Clinical Correlation

Malrotation with midgut volvulus should be considered in any neonate who presents with bilious emesis.

Key Points

- Midgut volvulus refers to a twisting of the bowel and mesentery, which occur when the normal attachments that anchor the bowel are absent or malformed. Compromise of the mesenteric vasculature and resultant bowel ischemia or infarction can quickly lead to shock or death.

- Neonates with no other obvious cause of bilious emesis require an emergent upper GI fluoroscopic study to expedite identification and treatment.

Midgut Volvulus on Radiograph vs. Fluoroscopy

Imaging in a patient with intestinal malrotation and midgut volvulus.

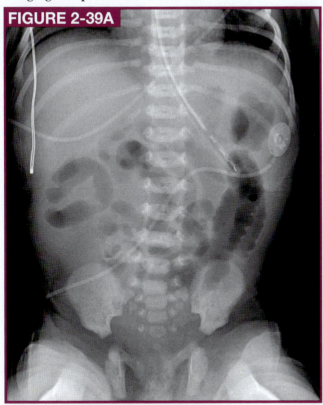

FIGURE 2-39A

An abdominal radiograph reveals a nonspecific, nonobstructive bowel gas pattern. Bowel loops have a somewhat tubular morphology, but there is no frank bowel dilation, pneumatosis intestinalis, or pneumoperitoneum.

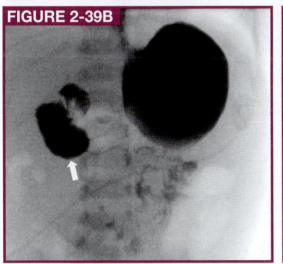

FIGURE 2-39B

Frontal view from a follow-up upper GI study reveals only minimal dilation of the proximal duodenum (arrow).

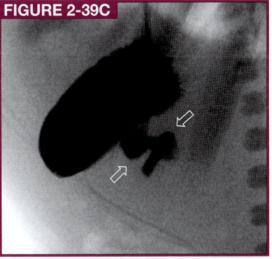

FIGURE 2-39C

The lateral fluoroscopic view shows the characteristic corkscrew appearance of the distal duodenum due to twisting of the bowel (arrows).

Jejunal Atresia

Imaging Findings

Gastric distension and proximal small bowel dilation will be present in jejunal atresia. The small number of dilated loops is more suggestive of a proximal small bowel obstruction than a distal small bowel or colonic obstruction.

Clinical Correlation

Patients with jejunal atresia develop abdominal distension and bilious vomiting within the first two days of life. Many infants with a proximal bowel obstruction will still pass meconium from the distal bowel segments, even if passage from the proximal bowel segments is delayed or completely blocked.

Key Points

- Jejunal atresia is thought to be secondary to a vascular disruption that results in bowel necrosis and resorption *in utero*. It has a low association with genetic abnormalities, but may be present in association with *in utero* midgut volvulus, gastroschisis, or thrombophilia.

- A contrast enema performed under fluoroscopy will help to evaluate for more distal causes of bowel obstruction in preparation for surgical intervention.

Jejunal Atresia Without Stomach Distension

FIGURE 2-40

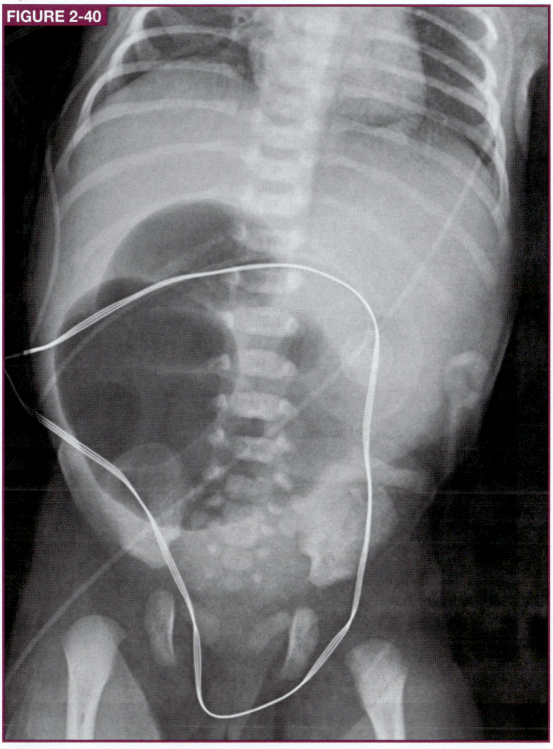

This abdominal radiograph of a neonate with jejunal atresia shows marked dilation of proximal bowel loops. The stomach is less distended in this image than is seen in typical cases.

Distal Bowel Obstruction

Imaging Findings

Distal bowel obstruction, which could be anatomic or functional, is indicated by multiple dilated bowel loops that extend into the distal small bowel or colon in a neonate with abdominal distension and vomiting. A contrast enema will help distinguish between the various causes of neonatal distal bowel obstruction. These include distal small bowel (ileal) atresia, meconium ileus associated with cystic fibrosis, meconium plug syndrome, neonatal small left colon syndrome (often associated with maternal gestational diabetes), and Hirschsprung's disease.

Clinical Correlation

A variety of abnormalities that cause distal bowel obstruction tend to present in a similar fashion – bilious vomiting, distended abdomen, and abnormal passage of meconium or stool. Surgery is required to repair bowel atresia and rectal suction biopsy is often performed in cases of suspected Hirschsprung's disease.

Key Points

- A water-soluble contrast enema can be therapeutic and curative in cases of meconium plug syndrome and neonatal small left colon syndrome.

- In many patients, a contrast enema will demonstrate a microcolon in the unused portion of the large bowel.

- It can be very difficult to distinguish small bowel from large bowel in a neonatal radiograph. The number of bowel loops that are dilated, rather than the morphological appearance, usually indicates that a distal obstruction is present.

Distal Bowel Obstruction With Dilated Bowel Loops

Abdominal radiographs in three neonates with distal bowel obstruction. Differential diagnosis includes distal small bowel (ileal) atresia, meconium ileus associated with cystic fibrosis, meconium plug syndrome, neonatal small left colon syndrome (often associated with maternal gestational diabetes), and Hirschsprung's disease.

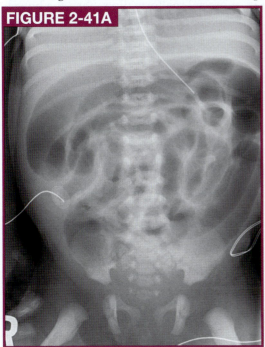

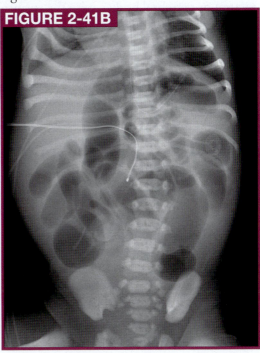

Multiple gas-filled loops of dilated bowel are present throughout the abdomen. In both cases, the stomach has been decompressed by an enteric tube.

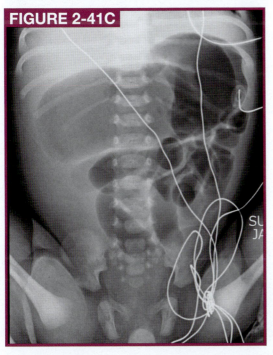

This image shows dilated bowel loops throughout the abdomen, as well as a dilated gas-filled stomach. An enteric tube has not yet been placed.

Imperforate Anus/Anorectal Malformation

Imaging Findings

Imperforate anus may appear similar to other causes of distal bowel obstruction on radiograph, with multiple dilated loops of bowel throughout the abdomen. Abnormalities of the sacrum or vertebral bodies raise the suspicion of anorectal malformation when the bowel is dilated. Inspect carefully for other VACTERL associations.

Clinical Correlation

Infants with imperforate anus or anorectal malformation will reveal an absent, malpositioned, or abnormally sized anal opening during physical examination. Abnormal stooling is common.

Key Points

- Multimodality imaging with fluorosocopy, ultrasound, CT, and MRI helps to evaluate the anatomic abnormalities associated with imperforate anus and anorectal malformation. Pelvic genitourinary organs are frequently involved.

Imperforate Anus With Dysplastic Sacrum

FIGURE 2-42A

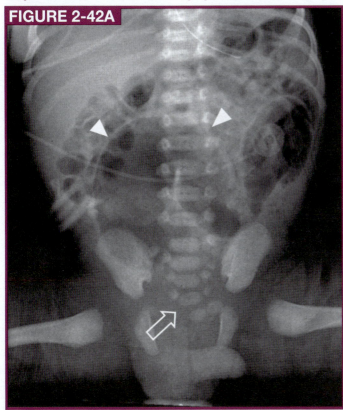

Dilated distal bowel loops (arrowheads) are seen on an anteroposterior abdominal radiograph of a neonate with imperforate anus. The dysplastic sacrum curves to the left inferiorly (open arrow). The stomach and proximal bowel loops have been decompressed with an enteric tube.

FIGURE 2-42B

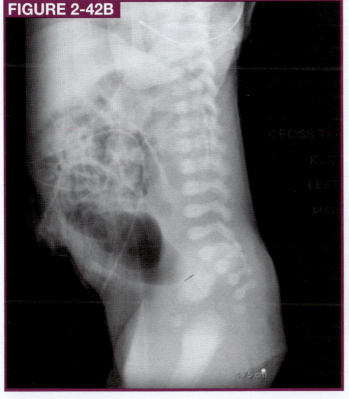

A cross-table lateral view was used to determine the distance between the blind-ending distal bowel and the skin surface. The distance between the gas-filled distal colon and the metallic BB marker placed at the expected anal opening measures 4.8 cm. A cross-table lateral view can also be acquired in the prone position for this purpose.

Anorectal Malformation With Dysplastic Sacrum

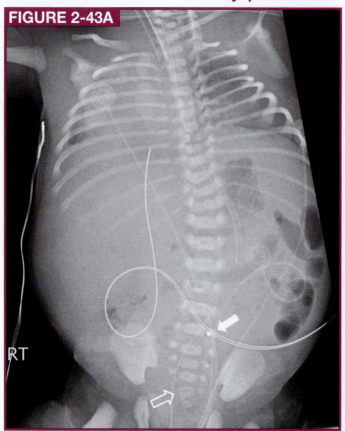

FIGURE 2-43A

This radiograph of another patient with anorectal malformation reveals decompressed bowel loops with an enteric tube in place and a dysplastic sacrum (open arrow). A BB marker placed under ultrasound guidance at the level of inferior termination of the spinal cord (closed arrow) projects at the level of the lumbosacral junction, which is too low.

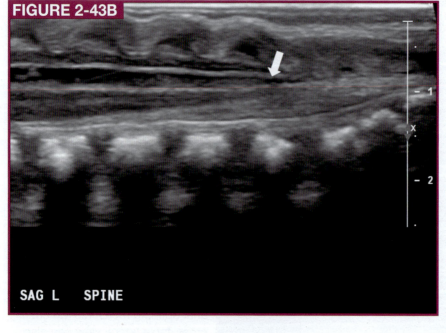

FIGURE 2-43B

An image from an ultrasound study of the spine shows low position of the spinal cord termination (arrow). The patient has a tethered cord and Müllerian duct anomalies.

Meconium Peritonitis

Imaging Findings

Meconium peritonitis results from *in utero* bowel perforation. It can manifest in many ways radiographically, including demonstration of gas- or fluid-containing abdominal collections (pseudocysts) that displace bowel loops or cause bowel obstruction. Occasionally, a contrast enema will reveal the site of perforation with extravasation of contrast into the peritoneal pseudocyst. Stippled or coarse focal or diffuse intraperitoneal calcifications frequently occur. These may be the only radiographic indications of bowel perforation.

Clinical Correlation

An abdominal pseudocyst may be detected on prenatal ultrasound. Neonates can also present with sepsis, bowel obstruction, or abdominal distension, prompting further imaging. Other times, calcifications may be found incidentally in patients with subclinical meconium peritonitis that has resolved on its own.

Key Points

- The presence of abdominal calcifications in a neonate should raise the possibility of meconium peritonitis. Other considerations include TORCH infections and vascular masses.

Meconium Peritonitis With Coarse Calcifications

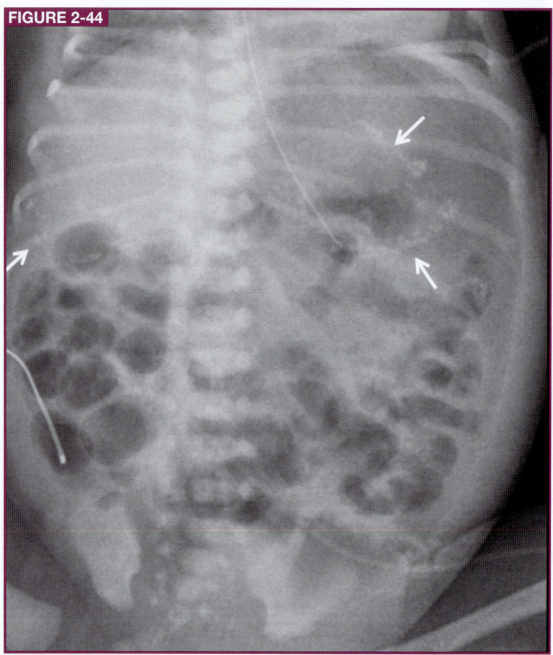

FIGURE 2-44

Coarse calcifications (arrows) are present in the upper abdomen of a neonate with meconium peritonitis. The large lucency over the left upper quadrant represents a contained bowel perforation with pseudocyst formation.

Meconium Peritonitis With Vague Calcifications

FIGURE 2-45A

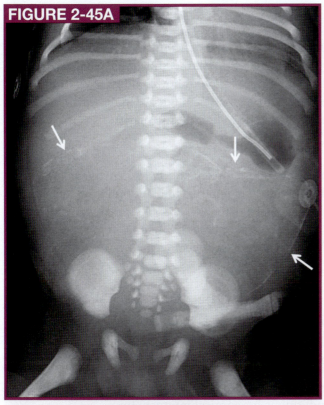

A frontal radiograph of the abdomen in an infant with emesis reveals vague calcifications over the mid- and lower abdomen (arrows) with a paucity of bowel gas. An enteric tube is in place.

FIGURE 2-45B

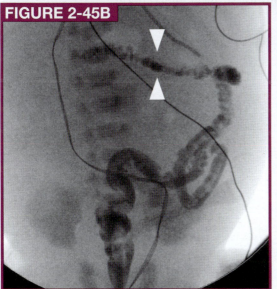

A follow-up fluoroscopic water-soluble contrast enema shows the small caliber of the colon, particularly at the level of the transverse colon (arrowheads).

FIGURE 2-45C

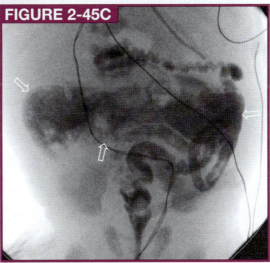

Further imaging demonstrates extravasation of contrast from the transverse colon filling a contained cystic space, known as a meconium pseudocyst.

Necrotizing Enterocolitis

Imaging Findings

Radiographic features of necrotizing enterocolitis are broad. They include specific findings of pneumatosis intestinalis, portal venous gas, and pneumoperitoneum; as well as nonspecific findings of bowel dilation, bowel wall thickening, separation of bowel loops, fixed bowel gas pattern, tubular bowel morphology, and ascites. To increase confidence in diagnosis, it is important to correlate the imaging appearance with the clinical presentation.

Clinical Correlation

Necrotizing enterocolitis is one of the most common neonatal abdominal emergencies. Presenting symptoms typically include bloody stools, vomiting, and abdominal distension, discoloration, or tenderness. Systemic signs of apnea, lethargy, or septic shock may be present. The disease is most frequently encountered in premature infants, but may also develop in neonates with congenital heart defects, hypoxic ischemic injury, or sepsis due to other causes.

Key Points

- Frequent serial radiographic examination is required to monitor the evolution of necrotizing enterocolitis and to evaluate for new findings, such as perforation.

- Left-lateral decubitus views help to evaluate for pneumoperitoneum in cases of necrotizing enterocolitis. Pneumoperitoneum or other signs of bowel perforation, such as loculated fluid collections, are indications for surgical intervention.

Necrotizing Enterocolitis With Pneumatosis Intestinalis

Two different patients with necrotizing enterocolitis demonstrate similar findings of pneumatosis intestinalis, portal venous gas, and tubular bowel loops.

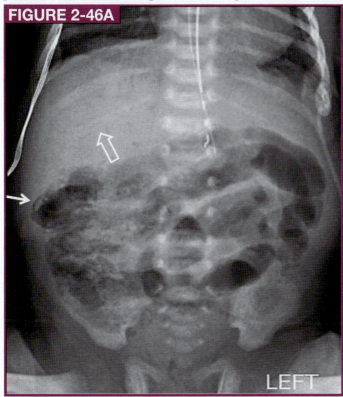

FIGURE 2-46A

Frontal view of the abdomen demonstrates small bubbly lucencies along the bowel walls, compatible with pneumatosis intestinalis (thin arrow). Portal venous gas manifests as small branching lucencies in the right upper quadrant (open arrow), where gas has drained from the bowel into the liver via the portal venous system.

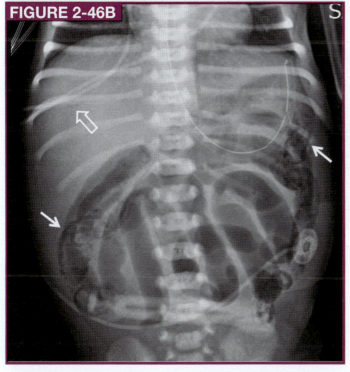

FIGURE 2-46B

In a second patient, there is even more extensive pneumatosis intestinalis (arrow). Portal venous gas is also present (open arrow).

Necrotizing Enterocolitis With Pneumoperitoneum

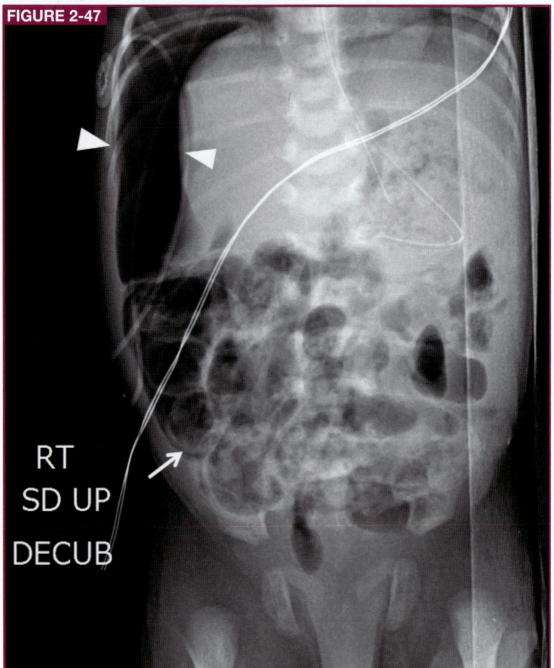

FIGURE 2-47

Another patient with necrotizing enterocolitis has mildly dilated loops of bowel, pneumatosis intestinalis (arrow), and pneumoperitoneum (arrowheads) evident on this left-lateral decubitus view of the abdomen.

Necrotizing Enterocolitis Totalis

Multiple views of the abdomen obtained in a patient with necrotizing enterocolitis totalis, who subsequently expired.

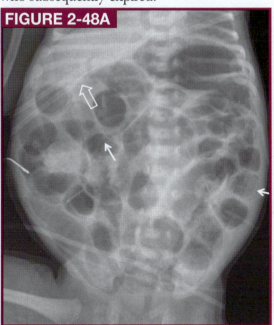

A supine frontal view of this premature neonate shows diffuse bowel dilation throughout the abdomen, extensive pneumatosis intestinalis (arrows), and portal venous gas (open arrow).

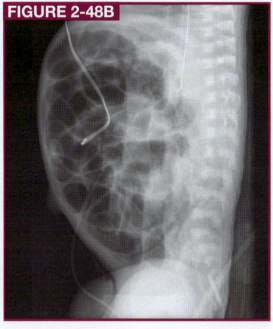

A cross-table lateral view demonstrates multiple fluid-fluid levels throughout the bowel.

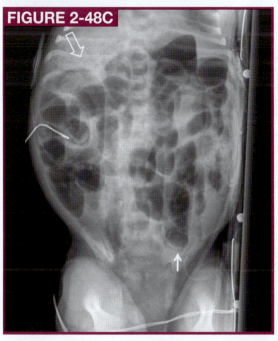

Pneumatosis intestinalis (arrow), portal venous gas (open arrow), fluid-fluid levels, and dilated bowel loops are also present on this left-lateral decubitus view. There is no pneumoperitoneum.

Necrotizing Enterocolitis With Bowel Wall Thickening

FIGURE 2-49

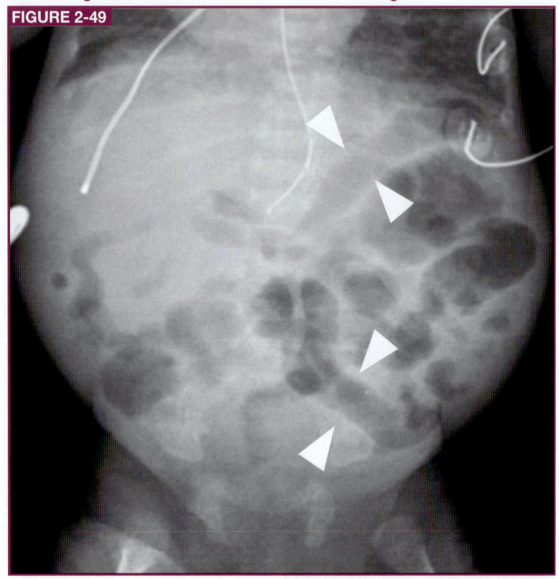

This abdominal radiograph of a premature neonate reveals clinical features of necrotizing enterocolitis. Tubular morphology of the bowel loops (arrowheads) and mild bowel loop separation indicate bowel wall thickening. No pneumatosis intestinalis, portal venous gas, or pneumoperitoneum is demonstrated. Note the interstitial changes of surfactant deficiency at the lung bases.

Necrotizing Enterocolitis With Fixed Bowel Loops

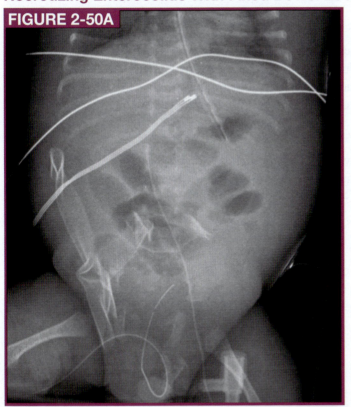

FIGURE 2-50A

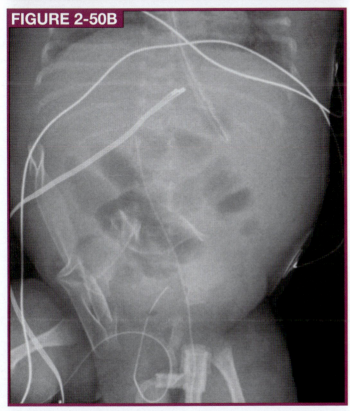

FIGURE 2-50B

These frontal radiographs of the abdomen, obtained nine hours apart, reveal a fixed bowel loop pattern indicative of infarcted bowel in a patient with necrotizing enterocolitis and a prior bowel perforation. A surgical drain, enteric tube, bladder catheter, and left lower-extremity PICC are in place.

Ascites

Imaging Findings

Moderate to large volumes of ascites cause centralization of gas-filled bowel loops in the abdomen as they float within the fluid. Interloop fluid may cause separation of bowel loops. Additional findings of pleural effusion, pericardial effusion, or body wall edema may be present with the third-spacing of fluid.

Clinical Correlation

On physical examination, patients with significant ascites will have abdominal distension with bulging flanks. There may be respiratory distress if the volume of fluid is great enough to restrict diaphragmatic expansion. Generalized swelling is often evident on visual inspection if third-spacing of fluid is present.

Key Points

- Ultrasound can be helpful in determining the presence, location, composition, and etiology of ascitic fluid. It can also be used to guide fluid aspiration for diagnostic purposes or symptomatic relief.

Ascites on Radiograph and Ultrasound

FIGURE 2-51A

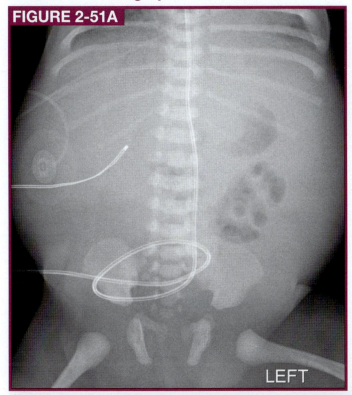

A neonate with ascites has a small number of gas-filled bowel loops in the central abdomen on radiograph. The abdomen is protuberant, with bulging of the flanks.

FIGURE 2-51B

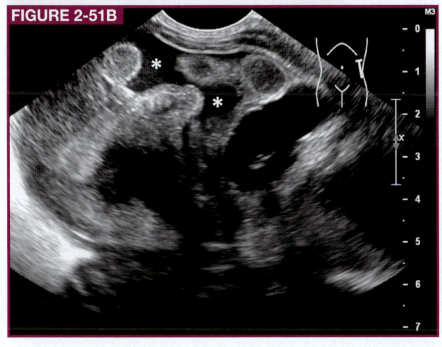

On ultrasound, ascites appears as anechoic areas located between the bowel loops and organs (asterisks).

Ascites With Fetal Hydrops

FIGURE 2-52

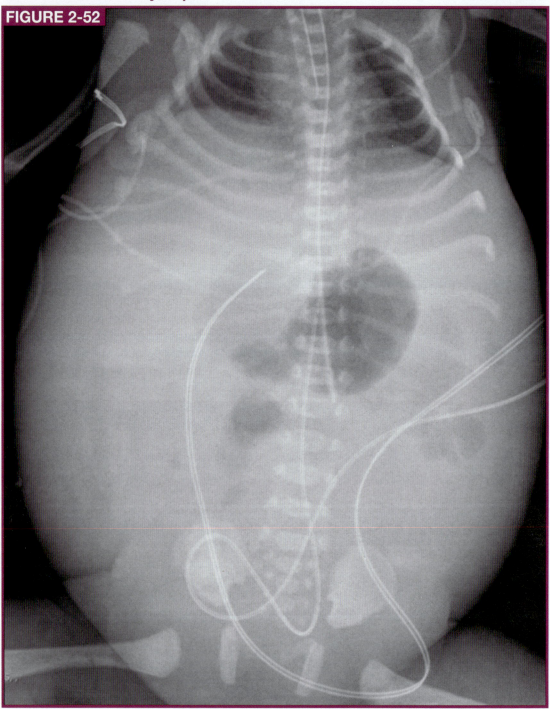

This frontal radiograph of a neonate with ascites and a history of fetal hydrops shows centralization of bowel loops, bulging flanks, small lung capacity due to mass effect on the diaphragm, and body wall edema.

Gastroschisis

Imaging Findings

Because diagnosis of gastroschisis is evident on visual inspection of the patient, imaging is not always performed in the immediate postnatal period. However, bowel loops will be seen projecting outside the abdomen if a radiograph is obtained. It may also reveal a scaphoid abdomen and paucity of intra-abdominal bowel.

Clinical Correlation

Gastroschisis is commonly diagnosed by prenatal ultrasound. On physical examination, the bowel and possibly other abdominal contents will be seen protruding through an anterior abdominal wall defect adjacent to the umbilicus. Unlike omphalocele, a membranous covering will not be present.

Key Points

- Long-term comorbidity in patients with gastroschisis results from bowel atresia, bowel obstruction, short gut syndrome, and bowel dysmotility. There is a relatively low association with genetic abnormalities, while infants with omphalocele have a higher incidence of associated syndromes and abnormalities.

Gastroschisis With Herniation of Bowel

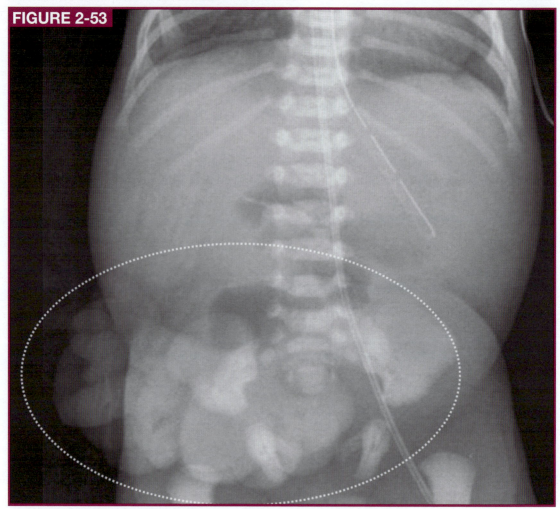

FIGURE 2-53

Air outlines bowel loops that have herniated through an anterior abdominal wall defect in this neonate with gastroschisis (dashed oval). The herniated bowel loops are mildly dilated and demonstrate wall thickening.

Omphalocele

Imaging Findings

On radiograph, omphalocele appears as a large soft tissue mass extending from the umbilicus. Gas-filled bowel can often be seen within the mass. As in gastroschisis, a scaphoid abdomen is usually present prior to correction, due to abdominal contents protruding through the abdominal wall defect.

Clinical Correlation

Similar to gastroschisis, omphalocele is evident on visual inspection of the patient and often diagnosed prenatally. It is distinguished from gastroschisis by its membranous covering and midline position at the level of the umbilicus. Larger omphaloceles (also known as giant omphaloceles) are generally more difficult to treat.

Key Points

- Although most cases of omphalocele are sporadic, they have a higher association with genetic anomalies, syndromes, and comorbid conditions than does gastroschisis.

- A correlation exists between pulmonary disease and the size of the omphalocele. Long-term pulmonary complications often persist after hospital discharge if a large omphalocele is present.

Omphalocele With Herniation of Abdominal Contents

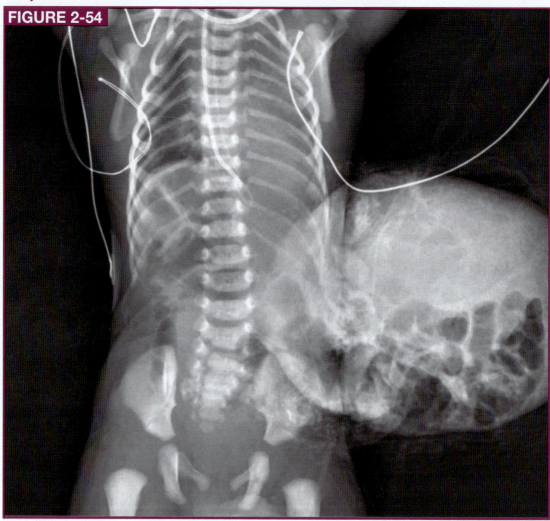

FIGURE 2-54

This supine abdominal radiograph of a neonate with a giant omphalocele reveals a soft tissue mass extending from the umbilicus and overlapping the left abdomen, which contains numerous gas-filled bowel loops. Soft tissue density along the superior aspect of the omphalocele is compatible with liver tissue. The small transverse dimension of the thorax and abdomen results from the herniation of abdominal contents into the omphalocele.

Omphalocele With Bowel Obstruction

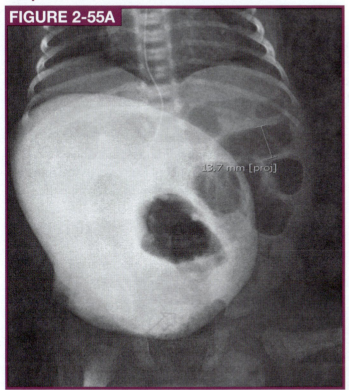

FIGURE 2-55A

Supine abdominal radiograph of an infant with omphalocele-related bowel obstruction shows gas-filled bowel within the omphalocele sac.

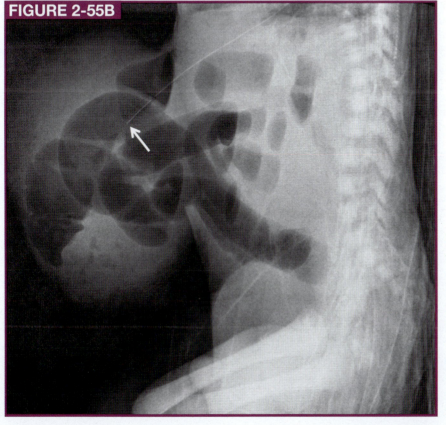

FIGURE 2-55B

Bowel loops are mildly dilated and demonstrate scattered gas-fluid levels on the lateral view. Note the enteric tube course, which extends into the stomach within the omphalocele.

Abdominal Masses

Imaging Findings

Large solid and cystic abdominal masses will push away surrounding bowel loops. There may be increased soft tissue density associated with the mass. Asymmetric rib expansion or chronic osseous remodeling indicate an underlying mass. Unless there is a calcified component, small masses are usually not evident upon plain radiography.

Clinical Correlation

Abdominal masses may present with abnormal prenatal imaging findings, palpable abnormality, or laboratory findings of organ dysfunction. Non-neoplastic masses are more common than neoplastic etiologies, but all require further investigation to determine the cause, guide management, and minimize long-term sequelae.

Key Points

- If an abdominal mass is suspected upon radiography or physical examination, an ultrasound should follow to determine the structure of origin and composition.

Abdominal Mass With Hydronephrosis

FIGURE 2-56

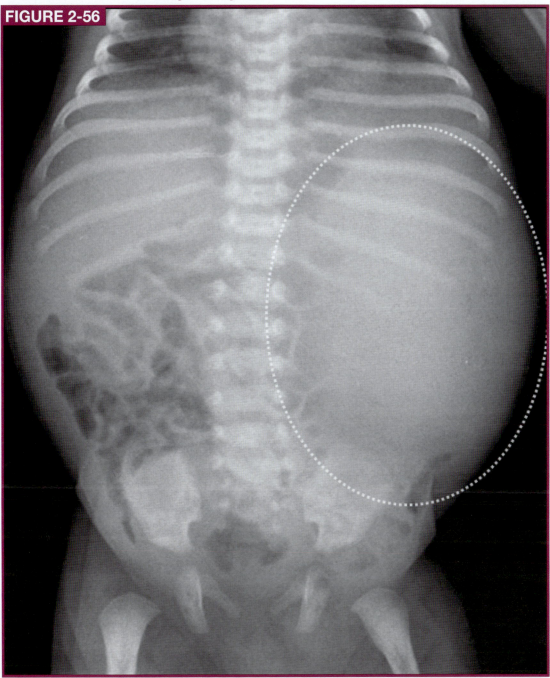

This abdominal radiograph shows a newborn infant with prenatal diagnosis of severe left-sided hydronephrosis. A soft tissue mass in the left abdomen represents the markedly enlarged left kidney (dashed oval), which is causing mass effect on the surrounding bowel loops.

Abdominal Masses With Hydrometrocolpos

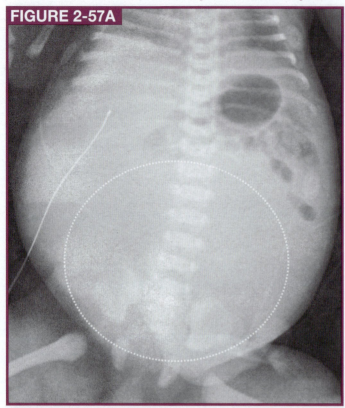

FIGURE 2-57A

Soft tissue density is seen in the lower abdomen of an infant with a palpable mass (dashed circle). There is associated superior displacement of gas-filled bowel loops.

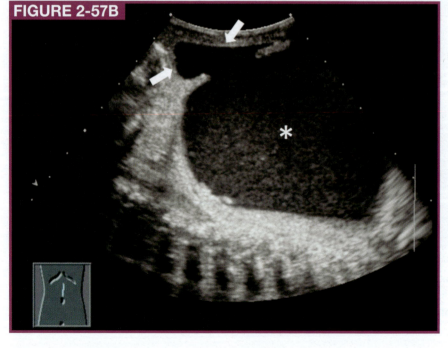

FIGURE 2-57B

Ultrasound examination reveals fluid dilation of the uterus (arrows) and vagina (asterisk) due to vaginal obstruction (hydrometrocolpos).

Abnormal Situs

Imaging Findings

Situs solitus refers to the normal position of the thoracic and abdominal organs. The cardiac apex should be directed to the patient's left lower chest. The gastric bubble should be seen in the left upper quadrant, and the liver shadow should project in the right upper quadrant. Any deviation from this pattern constitutes abnormal situs and should prompt further investigation to fully characterize the extent of anatomic abnormality.

Clinical Correlation

Situs abnormalities may be suspected in the setting of certain syndromes or by the presence of abnormalities detected on different imaging modalities, such as echocardiogram. Occasionally, patients remain asymptomatic and are found to have a situs abnormality incidentally after undergoing imaging as an adult.

Key Points

- Ultrasound helps to determine the position and orientation of the liver, as well as the presence of asplenia or polysplenia.

- Situs inversus refers to the position of the thoracoabdominal organs that is mirror-image to situs solitus. Situs ambiguous refers to cases in which there is abnormal position of the organs, but criteria for situs inversus are not met.

Example of Situs Solitus

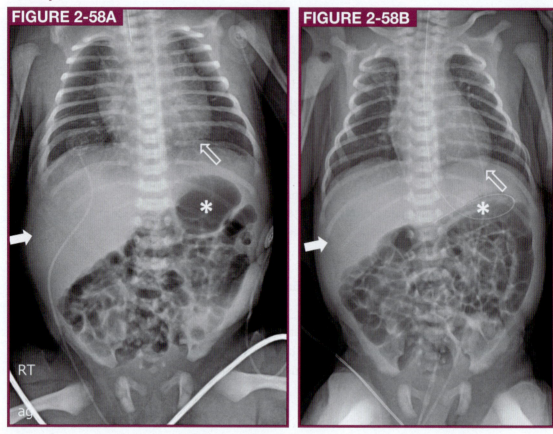

These radiographs show two different neonates with situs solitus. The cardiac apex is on the left (open arrows), the liver shadow is in the right upper quadrant (solid arrows), and the stomach is in the left upper quadrant (asterisks).

Example of Situs Inversus

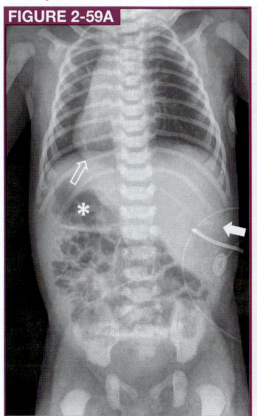

FIGURE 2-59A

Frontal view of the chest and abdomen in a patient with situs inversus. There is dextrocardia (open arrow), a left upper-quadrant liver (sold arrow), and a right upper-quadrant stomach (asterisk).

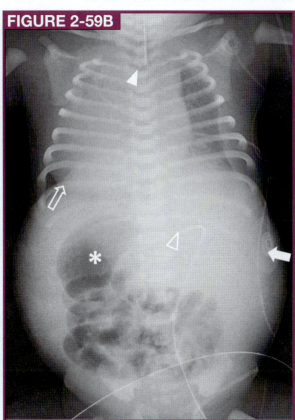

FIGURE 2-59B

A second patient with situs inversus also has dextrocardia (open arrow), a left upper-quadrant liver (solid arrow), and a right upper-quadrant stomach (asterisk). This patient also has ascites, cardiomegaly, and a malpositioned UVC (open arrowhead) and endotracheal tube (solid arrowhead).

Example of Situs Ambiguous

FIGURE 2-60

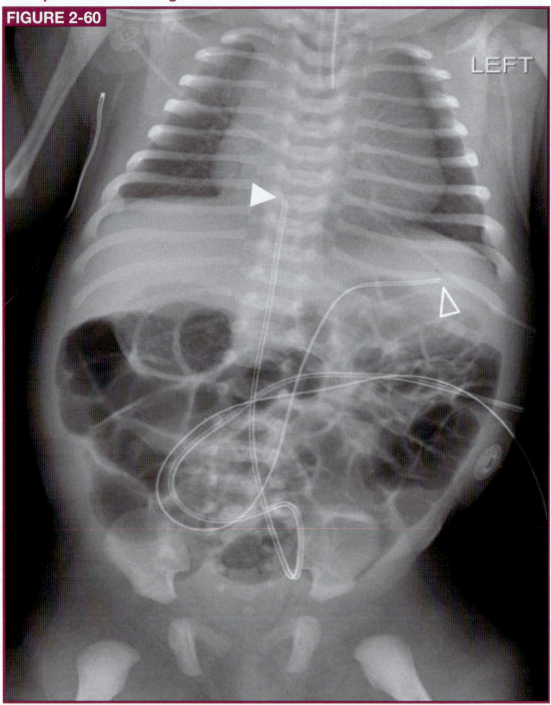

This patient with congenital heart disease has levocardia with transverse lie of the liver (situs ambiguous). The UAC courses slightly to the right of midline (solid arrowhead), overlying the right-sided aorta. The UVC is malpositioned (solid arrowhead), directed laterally and to the left over the liver.

Chapter 3 The Neonatal Head

TECHNIQUE

Ultrasound of the neonatal brain is performed primarily through the anterior fontanelle in the sagittal and coronal planes. Additional images are obtained through the posterior and mastoid fontanelles. Evaluation of the ventricular system, cerebrospinal fluid, and brain parenchyma is key to the diagnosis of intracranial hemorrhage, ischemia, and neonatal congenital malformations. The premature brain appears smooth and featureless because of underdeveloped gyri and sulci, which will gradually develop as the infant reaches term.

Head Ultrasound Technique

FIGURE 3-1

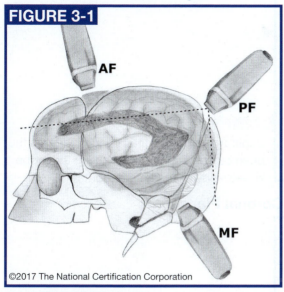

Ultrasound can easily be acquired through noncalcified portions of the neonatal skull at the anterior fontanelle (AF), posterior fontanelle (PF), and mastoid fontanelle (MF).

Neonatal Brain Survey

FIGURE 3-2

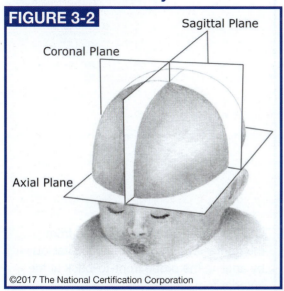

Coronal and sagittal plane images are frequently obtained through the anterior fontanelle. Axial and oblique axial plane images of the posterior fossa are primarily acquired through the mastoid fontanelle.

Anterior Fontanelle Approach to the Sagittal Plane

FIGURE 3-3

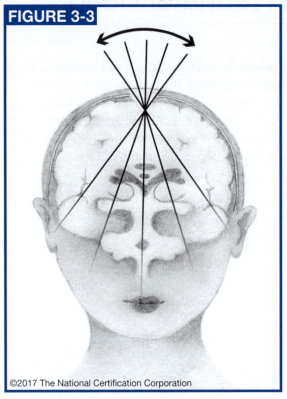

©2017 The National Certification Corporation

Sagittal and parasagittal images through the brain can be acquired by angling the probe side-to-side at the anterior fontanelle.

Anterior Fontanelle Approach to the Coronal Plane

FIGURE 3-4

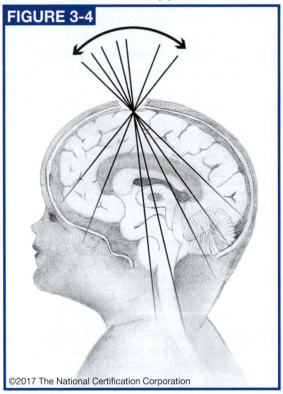

©2017 The National Certification Corporation

Coronal images can be obtained from the frontal lobe through the occipital lobe by angling the probe front-to-back at the anterior fontanelle.

NORMAL HEAD ULTRASOUND

Normal Head Ultrasound at Term

Multiple views from a normal head ultrasound of a term neonate demonstrate well-formed gyri and sulci and small, slit-like lateral ventricles. The choroid plexus is located at the roof of the third ventricle, along the medial margins of the body and atria of the lateral ventricles, and in the fourth ventricle. Normal choroid is the most echogenic structure in the brain and does not extend into the frontal or occipital horns.

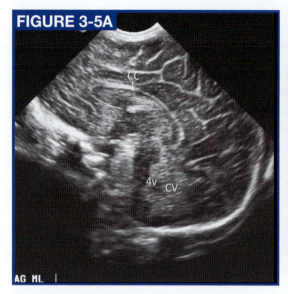

A midline sagittal view of the brain nicely demonstrates the normally formed corpus callosum (CC). The cerebellar vermis (CV) and fourth ventricle (4v) can be seen in the posterior fossa.

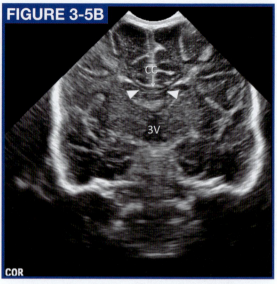

A coronal view of the brain through the level of the frontal horns shows the corpus callosum (CC) connecting the right and left cerebral hemispheres. The ventricles are slit-like (arrowheads) and the third ventricle is seen midline (3V).

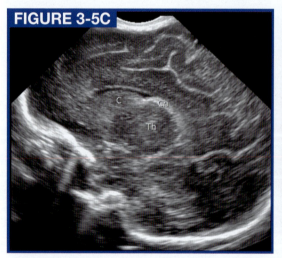

The left parasagittal view shows the head of the caudate nucleus (C) and thalamus (Th). The space between the caudate head and thalamus is called the caudothalamic groove, which is an important structure to evaluate for the presence of germinal matrix hemorrhage (GMH). The choroid plexus (Ch) appears as bright material within the lateral ventricle.

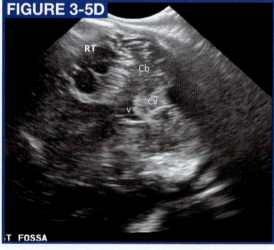

In the posterior fossa, the cerebellar hemispheres (Cb), cerebellar vermis (Cv), and fourth ventricle (v) are clearly seen on this view through the mastoid fontanelle.

Normal Head Ultrasound at 28 Weeks

This normal premature head ultrasound at 28 weeks demonstrates a smooth cerebral cortex, a faint echogenic periventricular halo of normal corticospinal tracts, and a small midline anechoic structure called the cavum septum pellucidum.

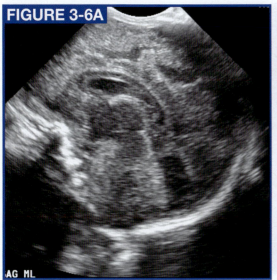

Midline sagittal view.

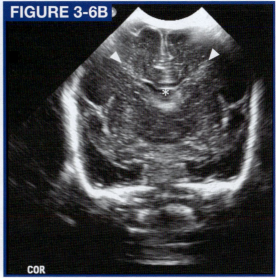

Coronal view. Note the small cavum septum pellucidum (asterisk) and faintly hyperechoic periventricular parenchyma (arrowheads), both normal findings.

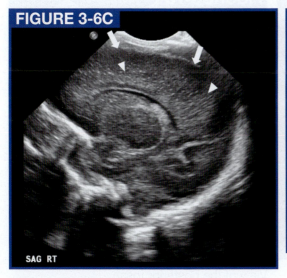

Right parasagittal view. The smooth cerebral cortex (arrows) and periventricular hyperechoic halo of cortical spinal tracts (arrowheads) are evident.

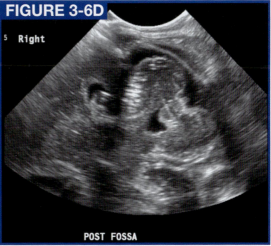

Mastoid view of the posterior fossa.

Normal Head Ultrasound at 23 Weeks

At 23 weeks gestational age, this head ultrasound demonstrates an even more prominent cavum septum pellucidum, extremely underdeveloped sulci and gyri, and larger ventricles vs. the 28 weeks and term examinations.

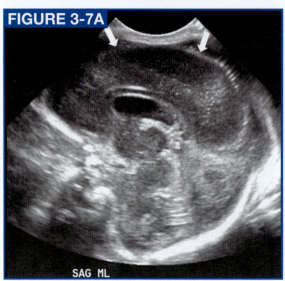

Midline sagittal view. Note the smooth brain surface (arrows).

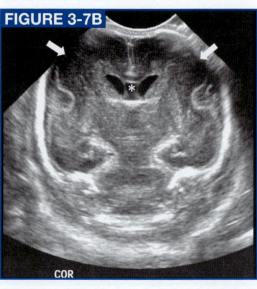

Coronal view. Note the smooth brain surface (arrows) and prominent cavum septum pellucidum (asterisk).

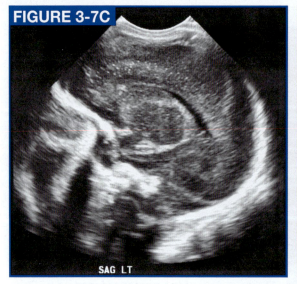

Right parasagittal view.

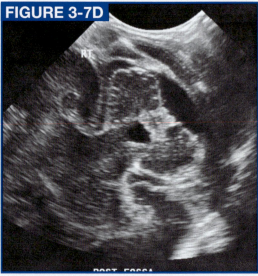

View of the posterior fossa.

PATHOLOGY

Germinal Matrix Hemorrhage (GMH)

Imaging Findings

A head ultrasound of a neonate with an acute GMH will demonstrate abnormal echogenic material at the caudothalamic groove. As the blood products age, they will become more hypoechoic. Intracranial hemorrhages are classified into four categories:

- Grade I is a hemorrhage localized to the germinal matrix at the caudothalamic groove only.

- Grade II demonstrates a GMH with extension into the lateral ventricle.

- Grade III demonstrates germinal matrix and intraventricular hemorrhage (IVH) with distension and dilation of the ventricular system by blood.

- Grade IV occurs when periventricular intraparenchymal hemorrhage develops due to venous infarction.

Clinical Correlation

Intracranial hemorrhage is common in preterm infants. Premature neonates are typically screened for GMH within the first week of life. If not diagnosed from screening, presenting symptoms may include decreased consciousness, hypotonia, seizures, low hematocrit, or apnea. The morbidity and mortality associated with GMH depend on the severity of the hemorrhage. Grade I and II hemorrhages usually resolve spontaneously with no clinical consequences. Grade III and IV hemorrhages are more likely to lead to long-term neurological sequelae.

Key Points

- The most common site of hemorrhage in premature infants is the germinal matrix, located along the caudothalamic groove. This area contains a high concentration of thin-walled vessels and is susceptible to stress in premature infants.

- Early identification of hemorrhage is important to ensure that supportive care is initiated in the acute phase.

Grade I GMH

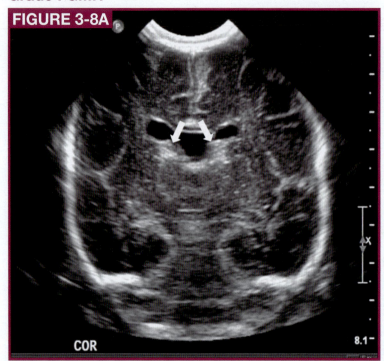

FIGURE 3-8A

Foci of echogenic material can be seen at the bilateral caudothalamic grooves in the coronal plane (arrows), compatible with grade I GMH.

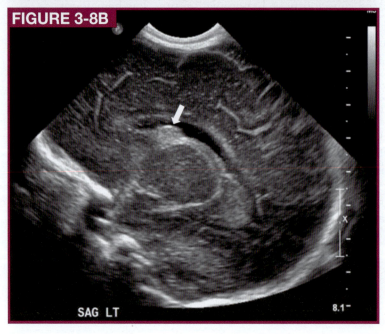

FIGURE 3-8B

In the left parasagittal view, the abnormal focus of increased echogenicity is again demonstrated at the caudothalamic groove (arrow), without extension into the ventricles.

Grade II GMH

FIGURE 3-9A

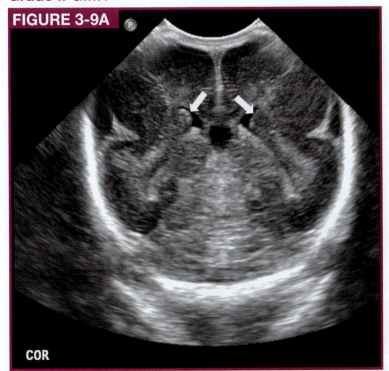

In this coronal image, the abnormal echogenic material extends from the caudothalamic grooves into the lateral ventricles (arrows), without development of hydrocephalus. Findings are compatible with grade II GMH.

FIGURE 3-9B

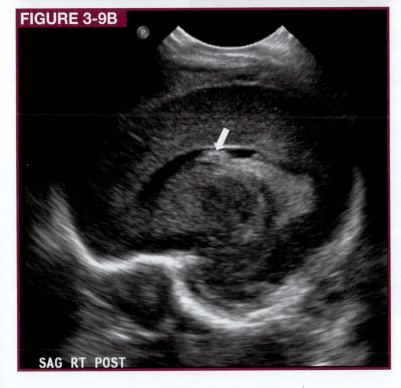

On this parasagittal view, abnormal echogenic material in the right lateral ventricle (arrow) represents blood products.

Grade III GMH

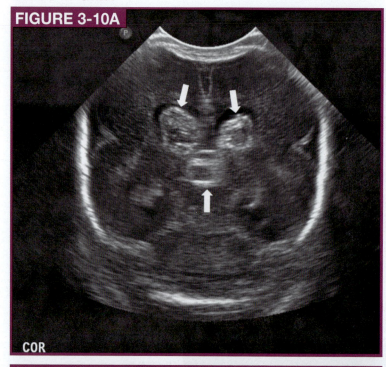

Echogenic blood products fill and distend the lateral and third ventricles (arrows) on the coronal image of a head ultrasound in an infant with grade III GMH.

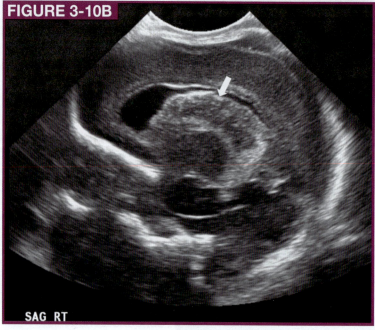

The right parasagittal view also shows hemorrhage nearly filling the lateral ventricle (arrow).

Grade IV GMH

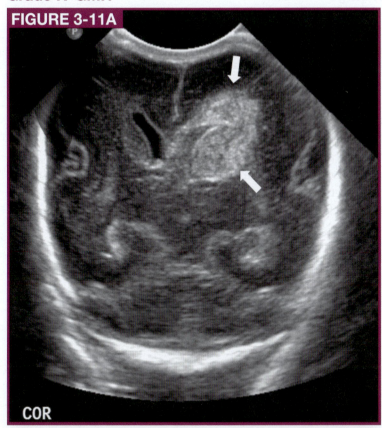

FIGURE 3-11A

A coronal view of the brain demonstrates intraventricular blood with hyperechoic areas in the left-frontal periventricular brain parenchyma (arrows), consistent with intraparenchymal involvement and grade IV GMH. The brain surface is very smooth due to extreme prematurity.

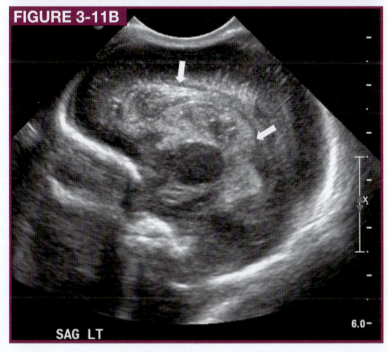

FIGURE 3-11B

Intraventricular and periventricular parenchymal hemorrhage (arrows) is also shown in this left parasagittal view.

Intraparenchymal Hemorrhage

Imaging Findings

Acute intraparenchymal hemorrhage on ultrasound appears as a well-circumscribed echogenic focus within the cerebral cortex, basal ganglia, or cerebellum.

Clinical Correlation

Intraparenchymal hemorrhage not associated with GMH is uncommon, but may occur under certain circumstances. Neonates on extracorporeal membrane oxygenation (ECMO) are at increased risk due to stress to fragile vessels caused by anticoagulation and hypoxia. Intraparenchymal hemorrhage can also occur spontaneously, secondary to thrombophilia, or as a complication of stroke or infection. Particular attention must be given to findings of mass effect and brain herniation, which can result in brainstem compression or obstructive hydrocephalus.

Key Points

- Although intraparenchymal hemorrhages occur less commonly than GMH, they carry a worse prognosis, with more severe neurological sequelae.

- Large intraparenchymal hemorrhages may develop acutely in patients on ECMO.

Intraparenchymal Hemorrhage in Right Temporal Lobe

FIGURE 3-12

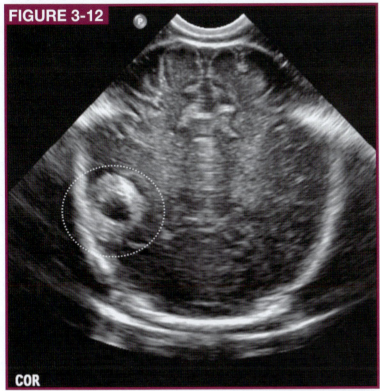

The focal, well-circumscribed hyperechoic area seen in this premature infant's right temporal lobe (dashed circle) is consistent with intraparenchymal hemorrhage. Most infants who develop intracranial hemorrhage on ECMO will be decannulated to avoid continued bleeding.

Intraparenchymal Hemorrhage in Right Cerebellar Hemisphere

FIGURE 3-13

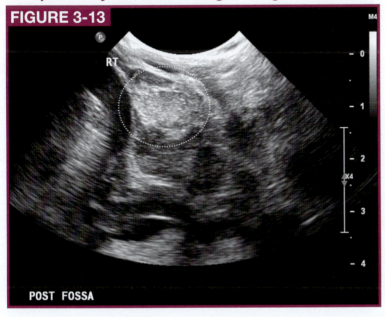

Images obtained through the mastoid fontanelle of a premature infant with dropping hematocrit demonstrate a hyperechoic focus within the right cerebellar hemisphere (dashed circle), consistent with intracerebellar hemorrhage.

Extra-Axial Hemorrhage

Imaging Findings

Like other types of intracranial hemorrhage, acute extra-axial collections are hyperechoic and become progressively hypoechoic as they break down. Subarachnoid hemorrhage extends along the gyri and sulci of the brain. Accurate differentiation between subdural and epidural hematomas is not always possible with ultrasound and is best assessed with MRI.

Clinical Correlation

Subdural hemorrhage is commonly caused by coagulopathy in preterm infants and by birth trauma in term infants. Common symptoms include seizure and hemiparesis if the hemorrhage is supratentorial, and apnea suggestive of brainstem compression if the hemorrhage is infratentorial. Careful evaluation for non-accidental trauma is warranted if no obvious cause is identified.

Key Points

- If a subdural hematoma or epidural hematoma is large enough, effacement of the gyri, midline shift, and compression of the ventricles may occur.

- Early detection can be critical to prevent brainstem herniation and death.

Subdural Hemorrhage

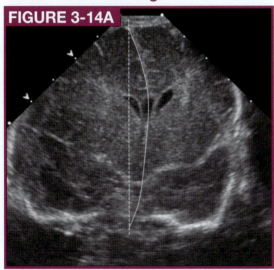

FIGURE 3-14A

A coronal view in a patient with subdural hemorrhage demonstrates right-to-left shift of the midline structures (solid line) from the normal midline (dashed line), indicating significant mass effect.

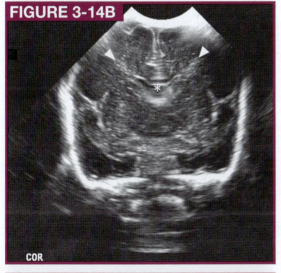

FIGURE 3-14B

A normal coronal view at a similar level is included for comparison. The small cavum septum pellucidum (asterisk) and faintly hyperechoic periventricular parenchyma (arrowheads) are both normal findings.

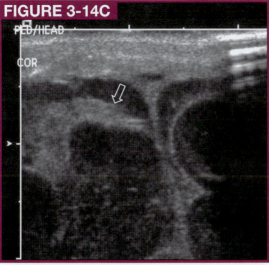

FIGURE 3-14C

A close-up coronal view obtained with a linear transducer reveals the echogenic extra-axial hemorrhage overlying the right cerebral hemisphere (open arrow).

Hydrocephalus

Imaging Findings

Hydrocephalus in neonates is usually the result of IVH or congenital brain malformation. Ultrasound examination will demonstrate enlarged ventricles. The number and location of dilated ventricles should be carefully evaluated to distinguish between communicating hydrocephalus (in which the interventricular channels remain open) and non-communicating hydrocephalus (in which obstruction of interventricular channels prevents the flow of cerebrospinal fluid), and to help identify the underlying cause.

Clinical Correlation

Clinical symptoms of increased intracranial pressure, such as apnea, stupor, vomiting, and bradycardia, may occur. Serial sonographic studies and ventricular measurements are often obtained in neonates with hydrocephalus to asses the need for shunt placement.

Key Points

- As the hemorrhage evolves, blood products will prevent the normal resorption of cerebrospinal fluid and may cause continued ventricular enlargement over time.

- Early identification of hydrocephalus is critical to assess the need for shunt placement and to minimize long-term sequelae.

Hydrocephalus at Seven Days of Age

Head ultrasound obtained on day of life seven in a preterm, extremely low birth weight (ELBW) infant born at 25 weeks gestational age demonstrates a grade IV GMH with a right periventricular intraparenchymal component.

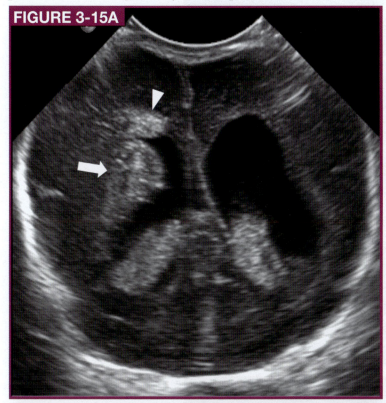

FIGURE 3-15A

The echogenic blood products can be seen within the lateral ventricle (arrow) and right periventricular parenchyma (arrowhead) on this coronal view.

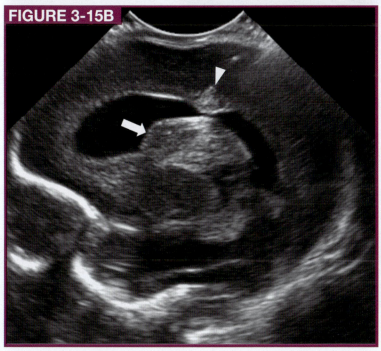

FIGURE 3-15B

Echogenic blood products are redemonstrated in the lateral ventricle (arrow) and periventricular parenchyma (arrowhead) on the parasagittal view. The intraparenchymal hemorrhage makes this a grade IV GMH.

Hydrocephalus at Three Weeks of Age

At three weeks of age, the infant's ventricular system has significantly dilated.

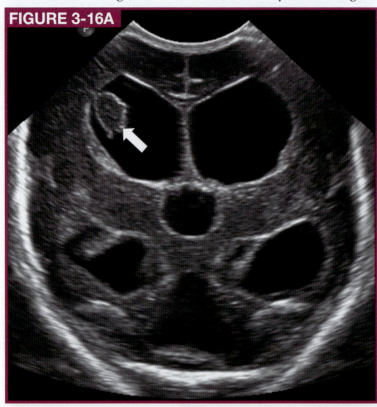

A blood clot is noted in the lateral ventricle (arrow) on the coronal view.

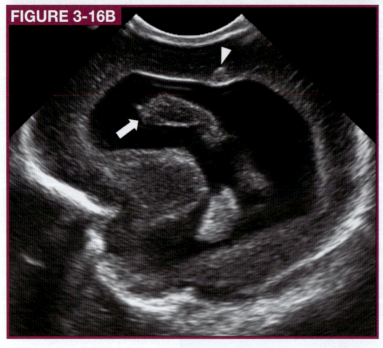

Evolving blood products are demonstrated in the right lateral ventricle (arrow) and periventricular parenchyma (arrowhead) on the parasagittal view.

Hydrocephalus at 4.5 Weeks of Age

At 4.5 weeks, the blood clot has nearly resolved. However, the ventricular system has progressively dilated, necessitating right-lateral ventricular shunt placement.

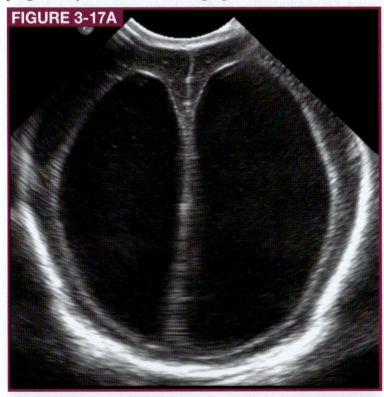

FIGURE 3-17A

The ventricles are severely dilated and occupy a large percentage of the intracranial compartment on this coronal view.

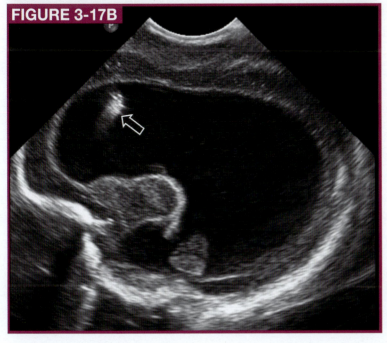

FIGURE 3-17B

On the parasagittal view, an echogenic focus representing the tip of the shunt catheter is seen in the frontal horn (open arrow).

Periventricular Leukomalacia (PVL)

Imaging Findings

Ultrasound of neonates with early PVL demonstrate increased echogenicity of periventricular white matter that is typically bilateral and symmetric. Over time, the periventricular parenchyma may become cavitary and multiple small cysts will develop. Larger areas of PVL are more likely to lead to cyst development. Encephalomalacia will occur in the later stages of PVL, resulting in parenchymal volume loss and enlargement of the ventricles.

Clinical Correlation

PVL and resultant encephalomalacia can result in severe neurological sequelae. Larger, more extensive areas of PVL are more likely to result in neurological deficits. Since the lower-extremity axons are in close proximity to the lateral ventricles, lower-extremity spastic diplegia is a common sequelae.

Key Points

- PVL can be confused with the normal periventricular halo. When compared with normal periventricular parenchyma, PVL tends to be more echogenic and brighter than the adjacent choroid plexus, with more well-circumscribed borders. The periventricular halo decreases in prominence when scanning through the posterior fontanelle, while the echogenicity of PVL persists.

Early PVL

FIGURE 3-18A

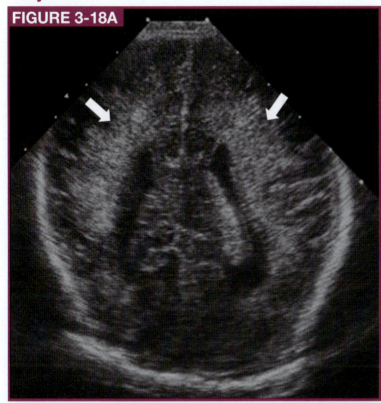

Initial coronal images from a head ultrasound performed at seven days of life demonstrate hyperechoic areas within the periventricular white matter that are symmetric and bilateral (arrows). This is consistent with early PVL.

FIGURE 3-18B

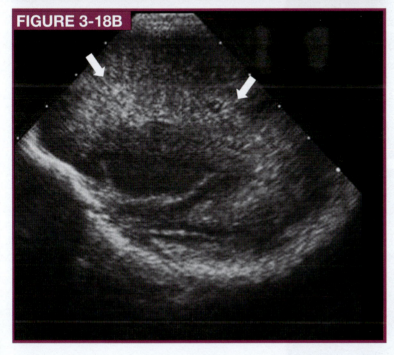

The hyperechoic parenchyma is well-seen in the parasagittal view (arrows).

Late-Stage PVL

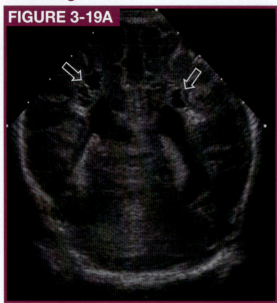

A coronal ultrasound image from the same patient several weeks later shows the development of multiple cysts surrounding the ventricles (open arrows) and associated parenchymal volume loss in the distribution of prior hyperechoic areas. Findings are compatible with evolving PVL.

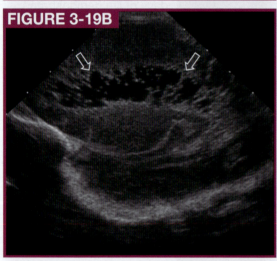

The cystic changes are well-seen in the parasagittal plane (open arrows).

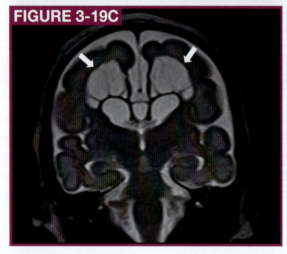

A subsequent MRI reveals large periventricular cystic spaces that are replacing the white matter (arrows).

Edema/Ischemia

Imaging Findings

Ischemic injuries in term neonates most commonly demonstrate imaging abnormalities in the more superficial frontal and parieto-occipital regions, as opposed to the deep periventricular lesions seen in preterm neonates. The most common findings are hyperechogenicity of the cortex, decreased corticomedullary differentiation, and poorly defined gyri and sulci due to resultant cerebral edema. In severe hypoxic events, the thalamus and basal ganglia will demonstrate increased echogenicity. Over time, encephalomalacia and ventriculomegaly may develop.

Clinical Correlation

There are many causes of neonatal hypoxic-ischemic injury, including asphyxia, sepsis, congenital heart disease, and trauma. Long-term clinical manifestations include dyskinetic and spastic cerebral palsy. Focal infarction can also occur and is more likely to lead to focal neurologic deficits.

Key Points

- Hypoxic-ischemic events in term neonates lead to decreased definition of the gyri and sulci and generalized increased echogenicity in the gray matter.

- The ventricles may appear small due to compression from cerebral edema.

Cerebral Edema in Term Infant

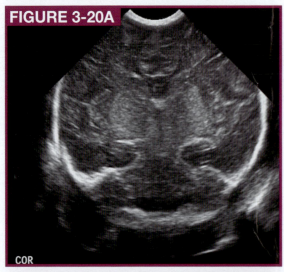

FIGURE 3-20A

Coronal view from a head ultrasound of a term infant after cardiopulmonary arrest reveals a generalized increase in echogenicity of the brain parenchyma with effacement of the sulci. There is poor differentiation of the gray and white matter. Note the small, slit-like ventricles.

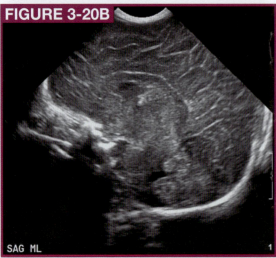

FIGURE 3-20B

The parasagittal view shows similar findings of increased parenchymal echogenicity, small ventricles, and effacement of the sulci.

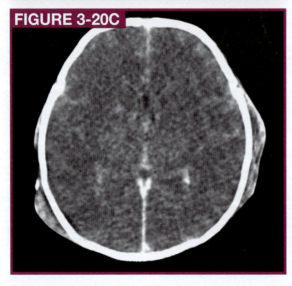

FIGURE 3-20C

A subsequent CT reveals diffuse cerebral edema with loss of gray-white differentiation, slit-like ventricles, and effacement of the extra-axial spaces. Subdural and subarachnoid blood products are also present, which are not clearly seen on the ultrasound images.

Lenticulostriate Vasculopathy

Imaging Findings

Ultrasound of a neonate with lenticulostriate vasculopathy will demonstrate echogenic linear structures along the vasculature of the basal ganglia bilaterally. Ventricular dilation, parenchymal calcifications, or cystic encephalomalacia may also be demonstrated if the vasculopathy is associated with a TORCH infection.

Clinical Correlation

Lenticulostriate vasculopathy is a nonspecific finding. In addition to TORCH infections, it may be seen in many other conditions, such as trisomy 21, fetal alcohol syndrome, neonatal hypoglycemia, and neonatal ischemia. It also occasionally occurs in healthy infants.

Key Points

- Lenticulostriate vasculopathy may indicate neonatal TORCH infections, congenital conditions, ischemic events, or it may be a transient normal finding in a healthy neonate. Further workup is necessary to determine the cause.

Example of Lenticulostriate Vasculopathy

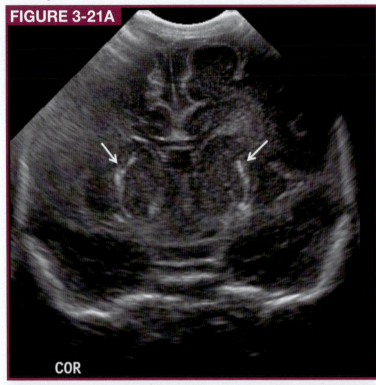

Coronal ultrasound images of a neonate with lenticulostriate vasculopathy demonstrate linear hyperechoic structures within the basal ganglia bilaterally (arrows).

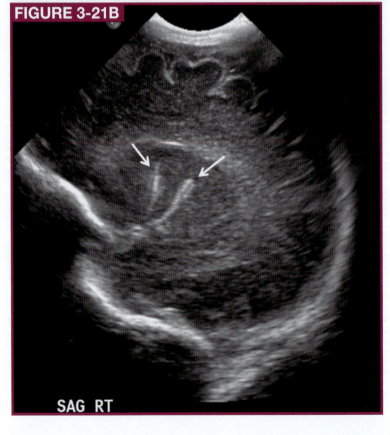

The hyperechoic vessels are seen coursing through the basal ganglia on the right parasagittal view (arrows).

Congenital Malformations

Congenital malformations of the brain can result from errors in development or insults to developing brain parenchyma. Malformations that lead to major macroscopic anatomic changes are detectable by neonatal ultrasound. However, a congenital malformation detected or suspected on neonatal head sonography should be followed up with an MRI of the brain for definitive characterization.

Choroid Plexus Cysts

Imaging Findings

Choroid plexus cysts appear as round anechoic structures in or along the choroid plexus of the lateral ventricles.

Clinical Correlation

Isolated or small choroid plexus cysts have no clinical significance, but cysts greater than 1 cm could indicate a chromosomal abnormality.

Key Points

- Choroid plexus cysts greater than 1 cm are associated with aneuploidy, particularly trisomy 18.

Insignificant Choroid Plexus Cyst

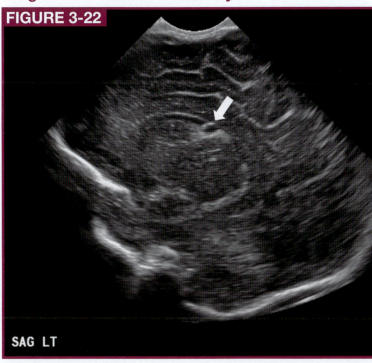

FIGURE 3-22

A small choroid plexus cyst measuring less than 1 cm is seen along the infant's choroid plexus (arrow). Choroid plexus cysts of this size are of no clinical significance.

Corpus Callosum Abnormalities

Imaging Findings

Antenatal and neonatal ultrasound can demonstrate partial or complete absence of the corpus callosum. Associated findings include widely spaced lateral ventricles with small frontal horns, absence of the septum pellucidum, a widened interhemispheric fissure, and dilation of the third ventricle.

Clinical Correlation

Dysgenesis or absence of the corpus callosum results from an insult during early gestation that leads to failure of the formation or migration of corpus callosum axons. It may occur in isolation or in association with other anomalies. Discovery should prompt close scrutiny of the remainder of the brain. Prognosis is extremely variable, but is more dependent on the associated anomalies than on the callosal dysgenesis itself. Therefore, partial dysgenesis and complete agenesis may be asymptomatic. Associated genetic syndromes may present with hypertelorism, dysmorphic facies, seizures, developmental delay, microcephaly, and other neurological abnormalities.

Key Points

- Corpus callosum congenital abnormalities have a wide spectrum of severity and clinical outcomes, ranging from partial dysgenesis to complete agenesis.
- Ultrasound evaluation is limited and MRI is necessary for complete characterization.

Corpus Callosum With Complete Agenesis

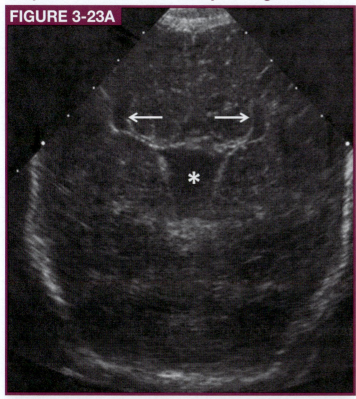

FIGURE 3-23A

The coronal image of a neonate with agenesis of the corpus callosum demonstrates a typical "moose head" or "longhorn" appearance of the frontal horns (arrows), with widely spaced lateral ventricles and dilation of the third ventricle (asterisk).

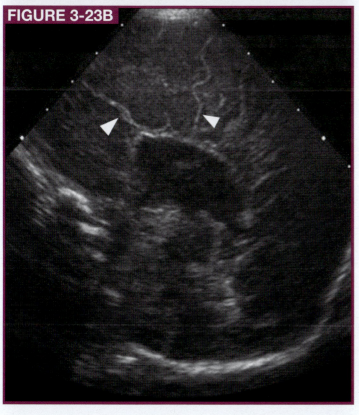

FIGURE 3-23B

The sagittal image demonstrates complete absence of the corpus callosum and adjacent gyri radiating toward the third ventricle (arrowheads).

Dandy Walker Malformations

Imaging Findings

Abnormalities along the Dandy Walker spectrum are the most common types of posterior fossa malformations. The classic Dandy Walker malformation includes hypoplasia of the cerebellar vermis, cystic dilatation of the fourth ventricle, and an enlarged posterior fossa; but a wide range of severity is seen along the spectrum. Dysgenesis of the corpus callosum is a frequent association.

Clinical Correlation

Neurological symptoms usually present within the first year of life. Macrocephaly is common. Although the anatomical abnormalities are in the posterior fossa, cerebellar symptoms are uncommon. Infants with Dandy Walker malformations have high mortality rates, especially if severe enough to be diagnosed antenatally. Cystoperitoneal shunts can help to decrease intracranial pressure in large malformations.

Key Points

- There is a wide spectrum of severity of Dandy Walker malformations. High morbidity and mortality rates are associated with severe malformations.

Example of Dandy Walker Malformation

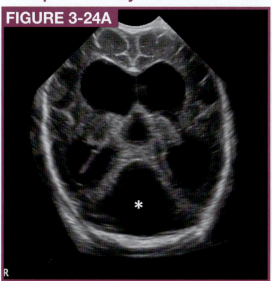

FIGURE 3-24A

A coronal ultrasound image of the brain reveals cystic enlargement of the posterior fossa (asterisk) and marked dilation of the lateral ventricles.

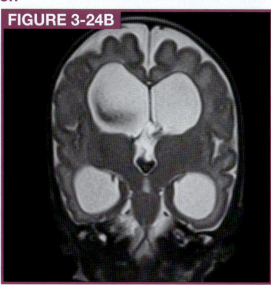

FIGURE 3-24B

A corresponding T2-weighted coronal MRI image of the brain also shows marked ventriculomegaly. Supratentorial hydrocephalus has occurred due to the compression of the cerebral aqueduct in the posterior fossa.

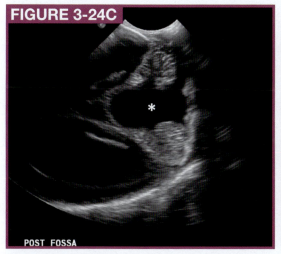

FIGURE 3-24C

An ultrasound image obtained through the mastoid fontanelle shows cystic dilation of the posterior fossa in communication with the enlarged fourth ventricle (asterisk). The cerebellar hemispheres are widely spaced, and there is vermian aplasia.

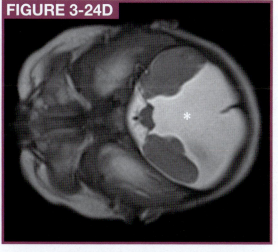

FIGURE 3-24D

A corresponding T2-weighted axial MRI image of the brain shows similar findings of cystic dilation of the posterior fossa in communication with the enlarged fourth ventricle (asterisk), widely spaced cerebellar hemispheres, and vermian aplasia.

Arnold Chiari Malformations

Imaging Findings

There are multiple types of Arnold Chiari malformations (also known as Chiari malformations), with type I and type II being the most common. Type I malformations result in caudal protrusion of cerebellar tonsils below the foramen magnum. Imaging demonstrates low-lying, pointed cerebellar tonsils extending through the foramen magnum. Type II malformations are more complex and include a clinically obvious myelomeningocele.

Clinical Correlation

Type I malformations are asymptomatic 50 percent of the time. Occasionally, headache, syncope, lower cranial nerve palsies, or neck and back pain may be presenting symptoms in an older child. Type II malformations have significantly higher morbidity.

Key Points

- Prenatal imaging of Arnold Chiari malformations help to determine the type of anomaly and associated abnormalities.

Arnold Chiari Malformation on Ultrasound

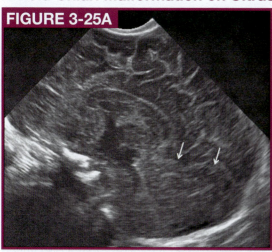

FIGURE 3-25A

A midline sagittal ultrasound image of the brain in a newborn with a neural tube defect demonstrates a small distorted cerebellum with crowding of the posterior fossa (arrows).

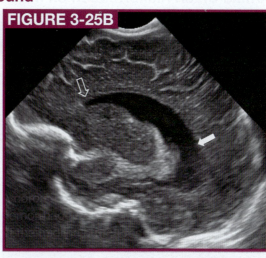

FIGURE 3-25B

A parasagittal ultrasound image shows findings of colpocephaly, including small, pointed, frontal horns (open arrow) and asymmetric dilation of the occipital horns (thick arrow) of the lateral ventricles.

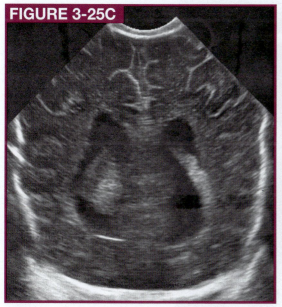

FIGURE 3-25C

A coronal ultrasound view of the brain shows dilation of the lateral ventricles.

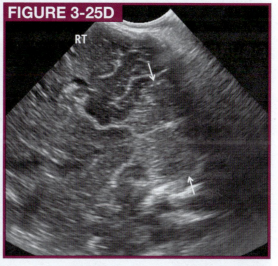

FIGURE 3-25D

In this ultrasound view of the posterior fossa, there is crowding of the cerebellum, which is small in size (thin arrows), with effacement of cerebrospinal fluid.

Arnold Chiari Malformation on MRI

FIGURE 3-26A

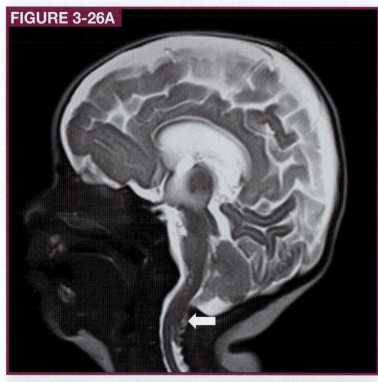

A midline sagittal MRI image of the same infant reveals inferior displacement of the cerebellar tonsils below the foramen magnum (arrow). The small posterior fossa is also demonstrated on this study.

FIGURE 3-26B

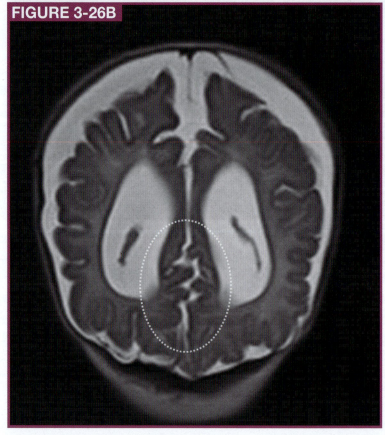

A coronal MRI image demonstrates lateral ventriculomegaly and interdigitation of the falx (dashed oval), which are frequently seen with type II Arnold Chiari malformations.

Arnold Chiari Malformation With Neural Tube Defect

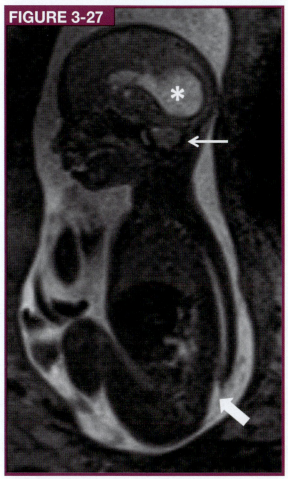

FIGURE 3-27

A fetal MRI obtained in a patient with a suspected neural tube defect shows a small posterior fossa (thin arrow) with inferior cerebellar herniation, ventriculomegaly (asterisk), and an open lumbosacral spinal dysraphism (thick arrow), which are also compatible with type II Arnold Chiari malformations. Obtaining the MRI before birth helps to confirm the diagnosis, characterize the location and severity of abnormalities, and evaluate the patient as a candidate for fetal intervention.

Chapter 4 The Neonatal Urinary Tract

TECHNIQUE

Neonatal kidney and bladder sonography is a frequently utilized and critical way to evaluate urinary obstruction, urinary tract infections, congenital anomalies, and renal masses. Ultrasound can provide superior image quality, which is usually sufficient to diagnose and follow common pathologies.

Three commonly used positions for ultrasound scanning of the urinary system include the lateral position, the prone position, and the pelvic position. Images of the kidneys and bladder are often acquired in both the transverse and sagittal plane.

Lateral Position

FIGURE 4-1A

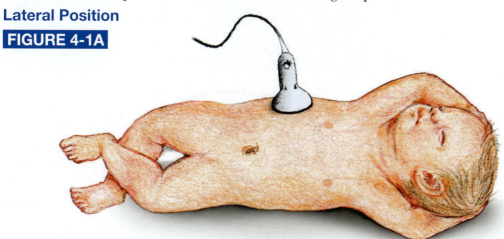

In the lateral position, the ultrasound probe is placed along the lateral aspect of the abdominal wall and flank at the level of the kidney.

Prone Position

FIGURE 4-1B

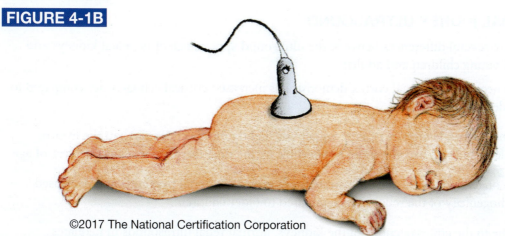

©2017 The National Certification Corporation

In the prone position, the ultrasound probe is placed along the flank posteriorly at the level of the kidney.

Pelvic Position

FIGURE 4-1C

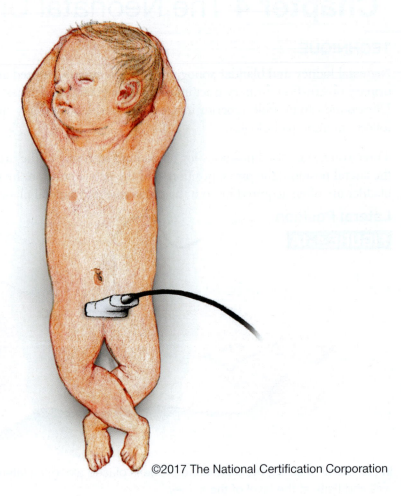

©2017 The National Certification Corporation

In the pelvic position, the ultrasound probe is placed in the suprapubic position midline.

NORMAL KIDNEY ULTRASOUND

There are several differences between the ultrasound appearance of neonatal kidneys and those of young children and adults:

- In neonates, the renal cortex demonstrates increased cortical echogenicity compared to older patients.

- The neonatal cortex is usually equally or slightly more echogenic than the liver or spleen and will become more hypoechoic by the time the child reaches one year of age.

- Neonatal kidneys also demonstrate more prominent renal pyramids and decreased echogenicity of the renal sinus compared to older children.

- Due to the embryogenesis of the kidneys, normal renal ultrasounds in neonates frequently demonstrate lobulation of the renal cortex. This is a normal finding, not to be confused with renal cortical scarring.

Normal Kidney Ultrasound
FIGURE 4-2

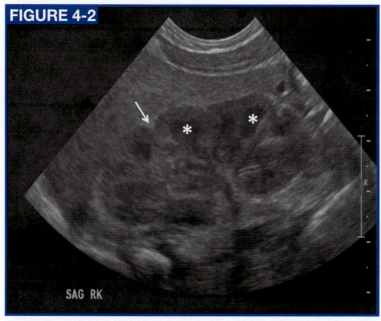

This normal sagittal ultrasound image of a neonatal kidney reveals the prominent hypoechoic renal pyramids (asterisks) and the slightly hyperechoic, lobulated renal cortex (arrow).

Normal Kidney Ultrasound With Minimal Sinus Fat
FIGURE 4-3

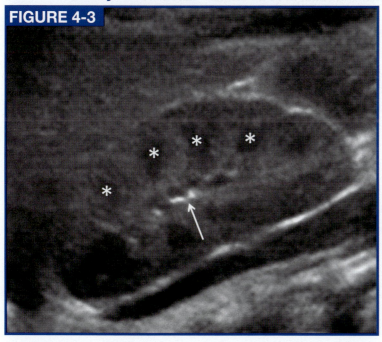

Another normal sagittal ultrasound of a neonatal kidney shows only minimal echogenicity of the renal sinus (arrow) due to the expected lack of renal sinus fat. Prominent renal pyramids (asterisks) are also noted.

PATHOLOGY

Hydronephrosis

Imaging Findings

Ultrasound of a neonate with hydronephrosis will demonstrate dilation of the renal pelvis and calyces to varying degrees. Although several classification systems are used in evaluation of hydronephrosis, this book will discuss the commonly encountered Society of Fetal Urology (SFU) grading system, in which:

- Grade 0 demonstrates no evidence of pelvic dilation.
- Grade 1 demonstrates mild dilation of the renal pelvis without dilation of the calyces.
- Grade 2 demonstrates dilation of the renal pelvis and some fluid in the calyces.
- Grade 3 demonstrates moderate dilation of the renal pelvis with uniform dilation and blunting of the calyces and normal renal parenchyma.
- Grade 4 demonstrates severe dilation of the renal pelvis and calyces with parenchymal thinning.

To aid in diagnosis and direct further management of hydronephrosis, be sure to note laterality, associated hydroureter, and changes in the urinary bladder.

Clinical Correlation

Congenital hydronephrosis is usually diagnosed on prenatal sonographic examination. Mild prenatal hydronephrosis may be incidental and resolve, but postnatal manifestations may include renal insufficiency, renal failure, or urinary tract infection. Severe hydronephrosis could lead to enlarged, palpable kidneys. Any significant compromise in prenatal renal function may lead to pulmonary hypoplasia.

Key Points

- There are multiple mechanical and functional causes for congenital hydronephrosis.
- Color flow images on Doppler ultrasound examination can help differentiate a dilated renal pelvis from prominent renal vessels.

SFU Grade 1 Hydronephrosis

FIGURE 4-4

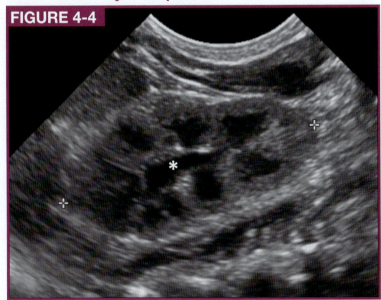

Sagittal renal ultrasound of a patient with SFU grade 1 hydronephrosis demonstrates mild dilation of the renal pelvis (asterisk).

SFU Grade 2 Hydronephrosis

FIGURE 4-5

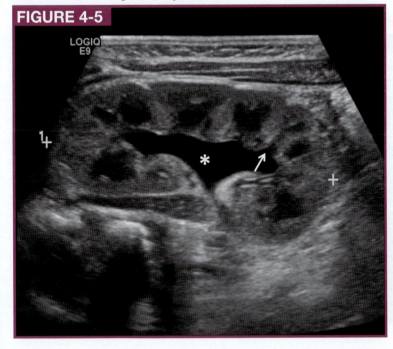

Sagittal renal ultrasound of a patient with SFU grade 2 hydronephrosis demonstrates moderate dilation of the renal pelvis (asterisk) with mild dilation of the renal calyces (arrow).

SFU Grade 3 Hydronephrosis

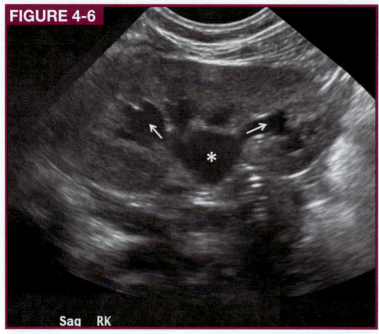

FIGURE 4-6

Sagittal renal ultrasound of a patient with SFU grade 3 hydronephrosis demonstrates moderate dilation of the renal pelvis (asterisk) and major and minor calyces (arrows), with normal renal parenchyma.

SFU Grade 3 Hydronephrosis Without Cortical Thinning

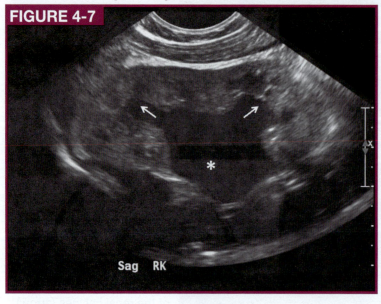

FIGURE 4-7

Another sagittal renal ultrasound of a patient with SFU grade 3 hydronephrosis shows severe dilation of the renal pelvis (asterisk) and calyceal dilation (arrows), but no evidence of cortical thinning.

SFU Grade 4 Hydronephrosis

FIGURE 4-8

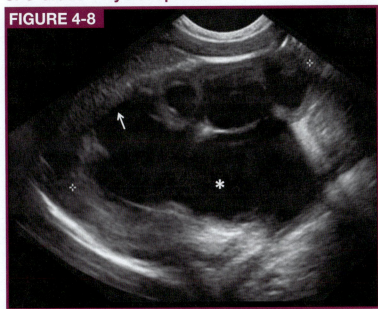

Sagittal renal ultrasound of a patient with SFU grade 4 hydronephrosis demonstrates gross dilation of the renal pelvis (asterisk) and calyces, blunting of the renal fornices (arrow), and parenchymal thinning.

Ureteropelvic Junction (UPJ) Obstruction

Imaging Findings

Ultrasound of a patient with UPJ obstruction will demonstrate multiple dilated calyces that communicate with a large renal pelvis. The ureter will not be dilated and the bladder will be normal. A severe obstruction may rupture the urinary collecting system, leading to urinoma or urine ascites.

Clinical Correlation

Intrinsic UPJ obstruction is thought to be caused by abnormal development of surrounding muscle. Retroperitoneal bands or adhesions are thought to be an extrinsic cause. Patients are usually diagnosed during prenatal ultrasound. Many patients are asymptomatic. Otherwise, neonates present clinically with a palpable abdominal mass and abdominal distension with abnormal renal function. Surgical treatment is most often required.

Key Points

- UPJ obstruction is the most common cause of congenital urinary tract infection.
- Nuclear medicine evaluation of renal function and obstruction helps to diagnose UPJ obstruction. Treatment is surgical.

UPJ Obstruction on Ultrasound

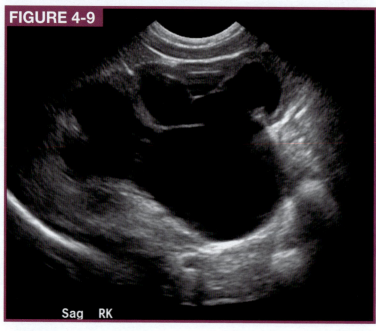

FIGURE 4-9

Sagittal ultrasound of a neonate with a UPJ obstruction demonstrates a severely dilated renal pelvis in communication with multiple dilated calyces and thinned surrounding renal parenchyma. There is no hydroureter.

Duplicated Collecting System

Imaging Findings

Depending on the degree of duplication, imaging findings of duplicated collecting systems will vary. In a complete duplication, two separate renal pelves and two ureters will be associated with the same kidney. The two ureters could join anywhere along the ureteral course, or may insert separately on the bladder in complete duplication. A bifid collecting system is also possible.

Clinical Correlation

Duplicated collecting systems occur when there is incomplete fusion of the upper- and lower-pole renal moieties during development, and lead to a variety of malformations. Symptoms are most likely to occur when there is associated vesicoureteral reflux or obstruction.

Key Points

- Classically with complete duplication, the upper pole ureter inserts in an ectopic inferomedial location on the bladder and the lower pole ureter inserts in the normal position. The upper pole is more likely to be obstructed, often from a ureterocele, and the lower pole is more likely to have reflux. Associated obstruction and reflux are not always present.

- Other modalities, such as fluoroscopy, MRI, or nuclear medicine may be utilized to fully evaluate anatomic and functional abnormalities if it is not possible to do so using ultrasound alone.

Duplicated Collecting System on Ultrasound and Voiding Cystourethrography (VCUG)

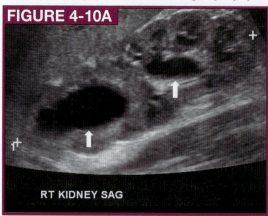

FIGURE 4-10A

A sagittal ultrasound image of the right kidney demonstrates a duplicated collecting system. There is hydronephrosis of the upper and lower pole moieties (thick arrows).

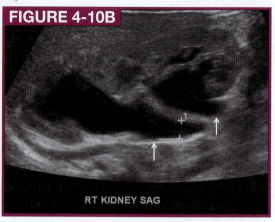

FIGURE 4-10B

This sagittal image acquired slightly more medially shows that each dilated collecting system has an associated dilated ureter (thin arrows).

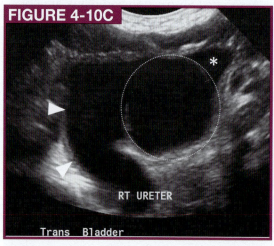

FIGURE 4-10C

The upper-pole moiety ureter (arrowhead) has an ectopic insertion on the urinary bladder and terminates in a ureterocele, which is the large cystic structure (dashed circle) occupying most of the bladder lumen (asterisk).

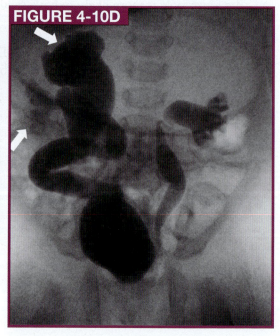

FIGURE 4-10D

A subsequently performed VCUG demonstrates bilateral vesicoureteral reflux. On the right side, contrast opacifies two separate ureters as well as separate upper and lower renal pelves (arrows).

Posterior Urethral Valves

Imaging Findings

Because posterior urethral valves lead to urinary obstruction, ultrasound findings commonly include bilateral hydronephrosis and hydroureter with a thick-walled, dilated bladder and dilated proximal urethra. The valve itself is not routinely seen by ultrasound. If the obstruction is severe enough *in utero*, renal dysplasia may occur, which manifests as small hyperechoic kidneys. Similar to UPJ obstruction, the renal pelvis may rupture, which leads to urinomas or urine ascites. VCUG is the test of choice to confirm diagnosis of posterior urethral valves postnatally.

Clinical Correlation

Posterior urethral valves are the most common cause of urethral obstruction in infant males. Prenatal ultrasound may suspect the abnormality. Clinically, infants may present with urinary tract infections, voiding abnormalities, renal insufficiency, or renal failure.

Key Points

- A posterior urethral valve is an abnormal mucosal fold or slip of tissue in the posterior urethra of male infants that leads to urethral obstruction. Over time, the muscles in the bladder wall will hypertrophy in response to outlet obstruction and increased intraluminal pressures. Ablation of the valvular tissue is required to relieve the obstruction.

Posterior Urethral Valves on Ultrasound

FIGURE 4-11A

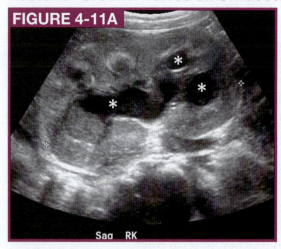

Sagittal ultrasound image of the right kidney demonstrates SFU grade 3 hydronephrosis (asterisks), one of the sequela of posterior urethral valves.

FIGURE 4-11B

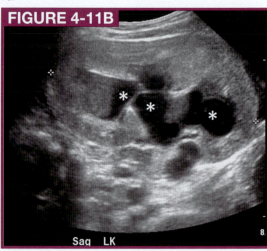

Sagittal ultrasound image of the left kidney also demonstrates SFU grade 3 hydronephrosis (asterisks). Bilateral hydronephrosis in a male infant is suspicious for the presence of posterior urethral valves.

FIGURE 4-11C

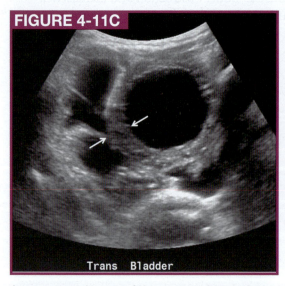

A transverse image of the suprapubic region demonstrates a thick-walled bladder (arrows), which is due to muscular hypertrophy in response to chronic bladder outlet obstruction.

FIGURE 4-11D

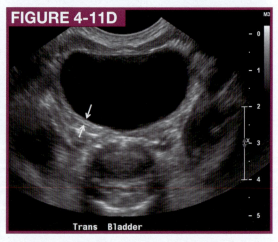

A transverse image of a normal neonatal urinary bladder included for comparison shows a thin, smooth bladder wall. The bladder wall should normally measure 3 mm or less if adequately distended.

Posterior Urethral Valves on VCUG

VCUG studies of three different male neonates.

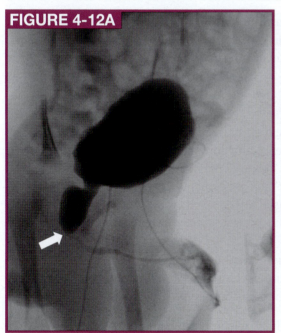

FIGURE 4-12A

Abrupt transition in caliber of the posterior urethra (arrow) with associated high-grade partial outlet obstruction is seen in a patient with newly diagnosed posterior urethral valves.

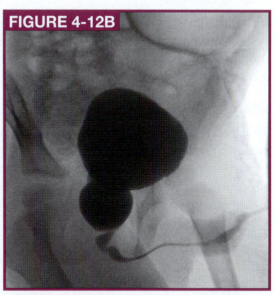

FIGURE 4-12B

A neonate after ablation of posterior urethral valves, with contrast flowing freely through persistently dilated posterior urethra valves. Dilation of the posterior urethra may persist after ablation.

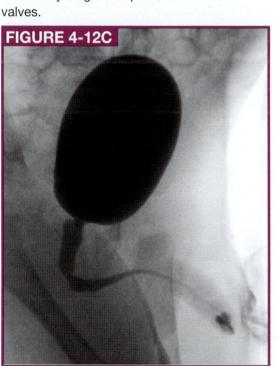

FIGURE 4-12C

A normal VCUG is included for comparison.

Multicystic Dysplastic Kidney (MCDK)

Imaging Findings

Ultrasound examination of MCDK will demonstrate multiple, non-communicating renal cysts of varying sizes with dysplastic renal tissue. The normal renal architecture is obliterated and the dysplastic kidney will usually involute over time. Compensatory hypertrophy of the contralateral kidney is expected.

Clinical Correlation

MCDK is related to abnormal renal development early in gestation. Diagnosis is usually made on prenatal ultrasound. Due to normal renal function, patients who are not diagnosed prenatally may never receive medical attention. Bilateral MCDK is almost universally fatal, but patients with a normal contralateral kidney have a normal life expectancy in the absence of other congenital anomalies or systemic disease.

Key Points

- Distinction between MCDK and severe hydronephrosis is critical to appropriately guide management. Communication of the cystic spaces indicates hydronephrosis rather than MCDK, and offers potential to preserve or gain some renal function.

- Careful evaluation of the contralateral kidney, which has a higher association with abnormalities such as reflux and ureteropelvic obstruction than the normal population, is required.

MCDK on Ultrasound

Sagittal ultrasounds from three different patients with MCDK demonstrate varying sizes of cysts and the dysplastic appearance of renal tissue. In each case, the cysts do not communicate with one another.

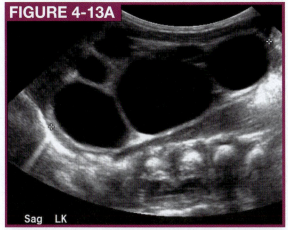

Large, non-communicating renal cysts are demonstrated in a patient with left-sided MCDK.

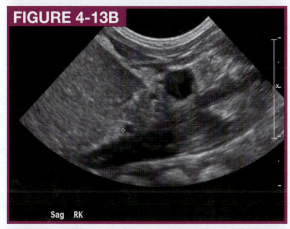

This image of the right kidney (marked with calipers) in a second patient with MCDK demonstrates small cysts of varying sizes and dysplastic echogenic renal parenchyma.

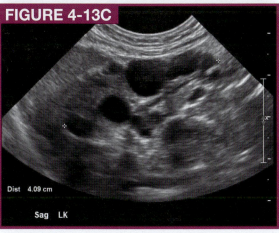

A third patient with MCDK has numerous non-communicating cysts of different sizes and dysplastic renal parenchyma in the left kidney.

Autosomal Recessive Polycystic Kidney Disease (ARPKD)

Imaging Findings

Ultrasound evaluation of a neonate with ARPKD will demonstrate enlarged, diffusely echogenic kidneys. Discrete cysts may not be evident until the patient becomes older.

Clinical Correlation

ARPKD is usually diagnosed during prenatal ultrasound. If not, neonates may present with palpable abdominal masses, pulmonary hypoplasia, hypertension, and renal impairment of varying severity. Although prognosis is variable, many patients will progress to end-stage renal failure and require dialysis or renal transplant. There is a high association of ARPKD with liver disease.

Key Points

- Autosomal dominant polycystic kidney disease is a separate condition which does not usually present in the neonatal period, although a diagnosis may be suspected based on a history of close family members with the disease.

ARPKD on Ultrasound

Renal ultrasound of a neonate with ARPKD demonstrates markedly enlarged and hyperechoic kidneys bilaterally.

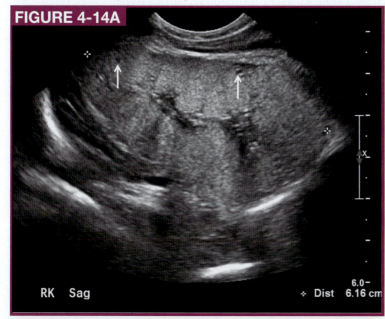

FIGURE 4-14A The right kidney measures 6.2 cm in length, enlarged for a neonate, and shows increased parenchymal echogenicity with innumerable tiny cysts (arrows) throughout.

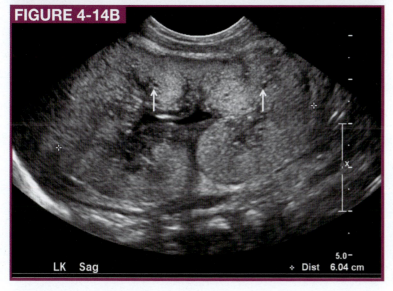

FIGURE 4-14B The left kidney is also enlarged, measuring 6 cm, and demonstrates similar findings of increased parenchymal echogenicity with innumerable tiny cysts (arrows).

Stasis Nephropathy

Imaging Findings

Stasis nephropathy (also known as Tamm-Horsfall proteinuria) causes hyperechoic renal pyramids bilaterally. The increased echogenicity may have a layering effect, but the central portion of the medulla is always involved. Segmental involvement can occur. Renal size and cortical echogenicity will be normal.

Clinical Correlation

Stasis nephropathy is typically seen in healthy term neonates. Accumulation of glycoproteins within the tubules can lead to increased echogenicity in the renal pyramids. Usually, patients are asymptomatic. However, transient renal dysfunction or oliguria may be present. It usually resolves in 7–10 days without treatment, but can persist longer in preterm infants.

Key Points

- Stasis nephropathy is a transient finding that is usually seen in healthy term neonates and is usually asymptomatic.

Stasis Nephropathy on Ultrasound

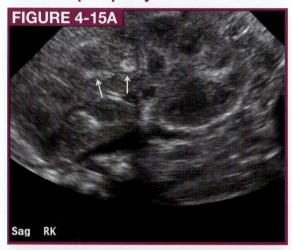

FIGURE 4-15A

A sagittal view of the right kidney demonstrates increased echogenicity at the tips of the renal pyramids (arrows). The kidney has abnormal corticomedullary differentiation, but is otherwise normal in appearance.

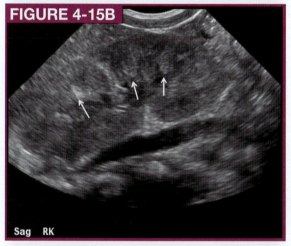

FIGURE 4-15B

An additional sagittal image of the right kidney acquired in a slightly different plane shows increased echogenicity of all the renal pyramids.

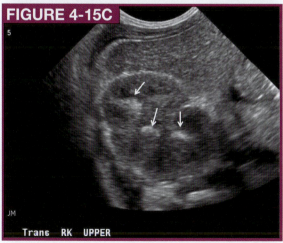

FIGURE 4-15C

The findings of increased echogenicity of the renal pyramids are reproduced in the transverse plane.

Adrenal Hemorrhage

Imaging Findings

Adrenal hemorrhage will manifest as a well-defined suprarenal mass involving either a portion of or the entire adrenal gland. Findings can be unilateral or bilateral. The hemorrhage will be hyperechoic in the acute phase, and will become increasingly hypoechoic as the blood products evolve. No blood flow will be demonstrated in the area of concern. The hemorrhage may resolve completely, or adrenal calcifications or cysts may remain as long-term sequelae.

Clinical Correlation

Spontaneous adrenal hemorrhage in term neonates is usually due to birth trauma, sepsis, hypoxia, or anticoagulation therapy. Although uncommon, patients may present with an abdominal mass or anemia. Adrenal insufficiency is a rare but potentially fatal complication.

Key Points

- Serial ultrasounds should be performed to ensure resolution and exclude the possibility of neuroblastoma.

Adrenal Hemorrhage on Ultrasound

FIGURE 4-16A

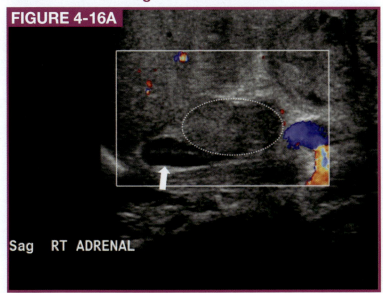

Ultrasound of a neonate with an adrenal hemorrhage demonstrates a mildly heterogeneous, well-circumscribed mass (dashed oval) partially encompassing the adrenal gland (arrow), with no evidence of internal vascularity.

FIGURE 4-16B

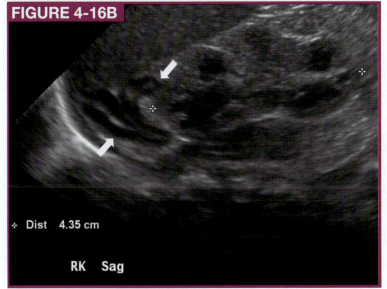

For comparison, the normal adrenal gland (arrows) demonstrates a thin, linear, Y-shaped organ at the upper pole of the right kidney. Clear delineation of the cortex and medulla creates a layered appearance, which has been likened to that of a sandwich cookie.

Chapter 5 Artifacts

Imaging artifacts are common and may confuse study results by simulating disease. The ability to recognize common artifacts is important in order to interpret images accurately. When in doubt, visual inspection of the patient or additional imaging may help to differentiate artifacts from true disease.

SKIN FOLDS

Skin folds can be very prominent and mimic pneumothoraces. Linear lucency that extends beyond the lung margin into the soft tissues of the chest wall indicates that the origin is outside the thoracic cavity. A true pneumothorax will have peripheral lucency that assumes a shape similar to the pleural space.

Skin Fold Mimicking Pneumothorax

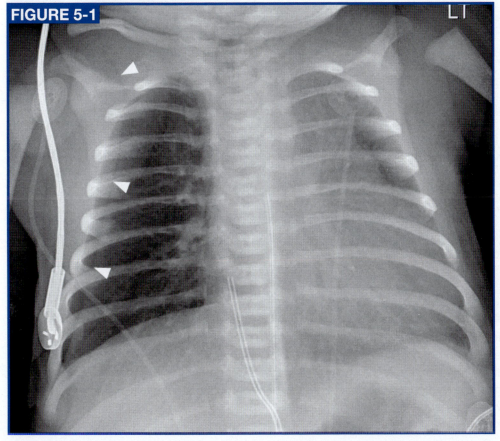

FIGURE 5-1

The skin fold along the right lateral chest wall in this infant (arrowheads) is very similar in appearance to a true pneumothorax. Careful evaluation reveals that the lucency extends outside the thoracic cavity superiorly. If the etiology of a thoracic lucency remains unclear, a follow-up radiograph obtained in the decubitus position (with side in question directed away from the table) can help to clarify.

Skin Folds Not Conforming to Pleural Contour

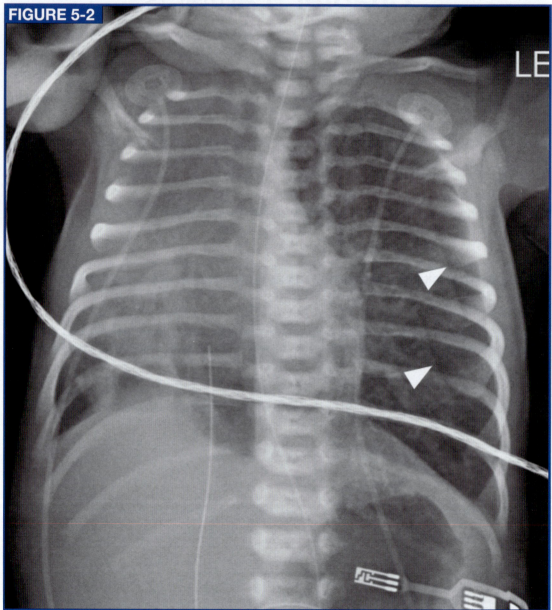

FIGURE 5-2

Two skin folds are seen in the left hemithorax of this premature infant (arrowheads). The shape of the lucencies do not conform to the normal pleural contour and lung markings are seen peripherally. In addition, the more superior skin fold extends outside the thoracic cavity, which is not compatible with pneumothorax. Note the near-complete atelectasis of the right lung, with rightward shift of the mediastinal structures.

MACH EFFECT

Mach effect results in an exaggerated lucency between two structures of different densities. In the chest, it most commonly occurs at the junction of the mediastinal silhouette and the lung parenchyma, simulating pneumothorax or pneumomediastinum.

Mach Effect With Lung Disease of Prematurity

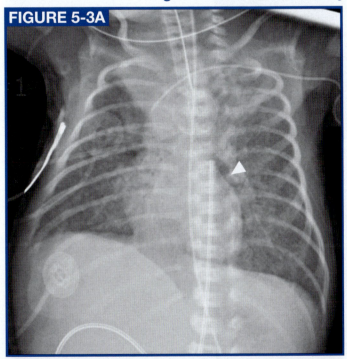

FIGURE 5-3A

The prominent lucency along the left cardiac border (arrowhead) is due to Mach effect.

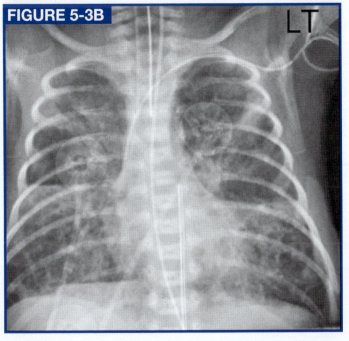

FIGURE 5-3B

A follow-up radiograph 24 hours later shows resolution of the lucency. Note the diffuse interstitial changes of lung disease of prematurity with migrating areas of atelectasis.

Mach Effect With Malpositioned Endotracheal Tube (ETT)

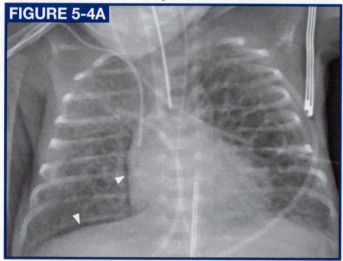

FIGURE 5-4A

A lucency due to Mach effect is seen along the right mediastinal border and lung base of another premature infant (arrowheads).

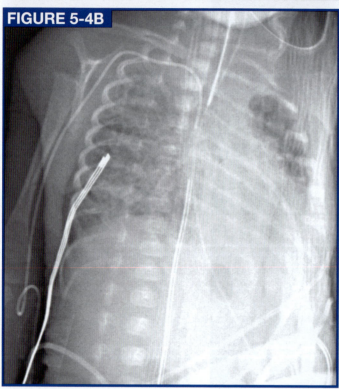

FIGURE 5-4B

A follow-up left-lateral decubitus view of the chest reveals no pneumothorax. Note the low-lying ETT in the initial image, which was adjusted prior to the follow-up examination.

MONITORING LEADS AND DEVICES

It is important to differentiate external monitoring leads and devices from support lines and tubes within the patient. Follow the course and position of the material in question to determine what it represents. It is helpful to correlate with visual inspection of the patient, when possible.

Example of External Monitoring Leads on Radiograph

FIGURE 5-5

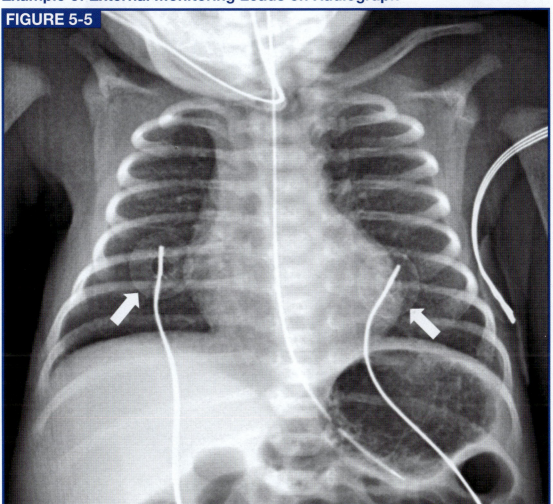

Telemetry leads (arrows) overlie the chest of this preterm infant. The vague round densities seen at the tips of the leads represent adhesive pads on the surface of the patient's skin.

Example of External vs. Internal Materials on Radiograph

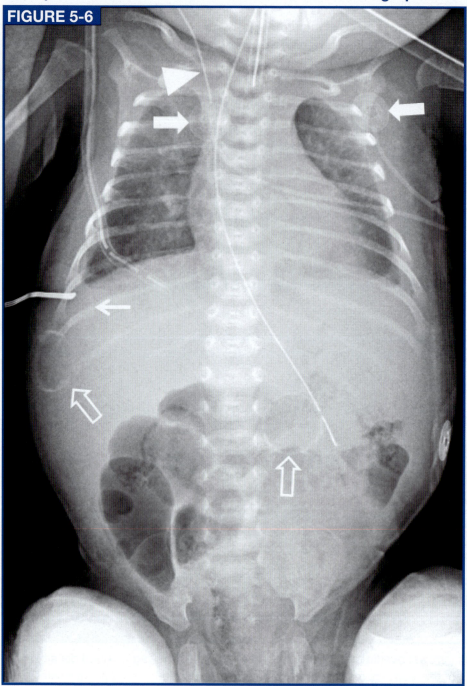

FIGURE 5-6

Two faint round densities projecting over the left-medial and right-lateral upper quadrants represent cutaneous carbon dioxide monitors (open arrows). A duck-shaped cutaneous temperature monitor overlies the right costophrenic angle (thin arrow). Telemetry leads project over the chest (thick arrows). An ETT, enteric tube, thoracostomy tube, and right scalp peripherally inserted central catheter (PICC) are inside the patient, who has pneumatosis intestinalis due to necrotizing enterocolitis. Note that it could be easy to mistake the right scalp PICC (arrowhead) as being in continuity with the overlying telemetry lead.

CLOTHING AND DIAPERS

Common items used to clothe the neonate can have unusual radiographic appearances. When possible, the patient should have all clothing and patterned fabrics removed prior to radiographic examination.

Diaper Simulating Mottling Over Pelvis

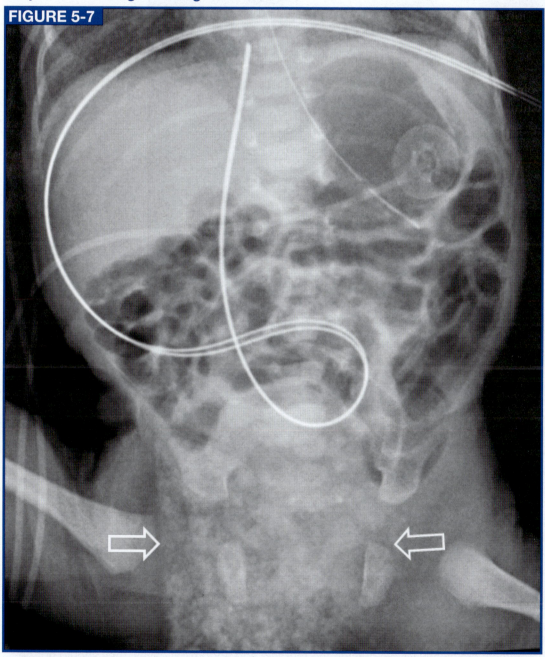

FIGURE 5-7

The mottled density projecting over the pelvis of this neonate (open arrows) is due to a wet diaper.

Clothing Potentially Obscuring Calcifications

FIGURE 5-8

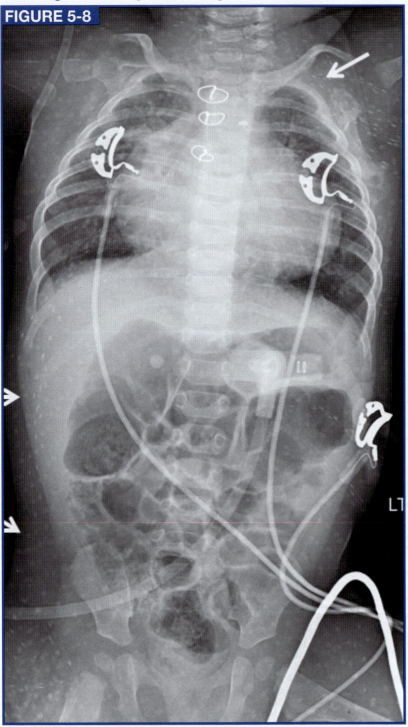

Tiny scattered round densities projecting over the chest, abdomen, and pelvis of this infant with congenital heart disease (arrows) are due to the pattern of the patient's clothing. Because the artifacts are clearly visible outside the thoracic and abdominal cavity, they should not be confused with disease, but could obscure evaluation of the lung parenchyma or calcifications. Note the median sternotomy wires, cardiomegaly, and gastrostomy tube.

COMFORT ITEMS

Toys, pacifiers, and other comfort items often used to console young children may obscure important structures or cause confusion if they overlie the patient.

Example of Plush Toy on Radiograph

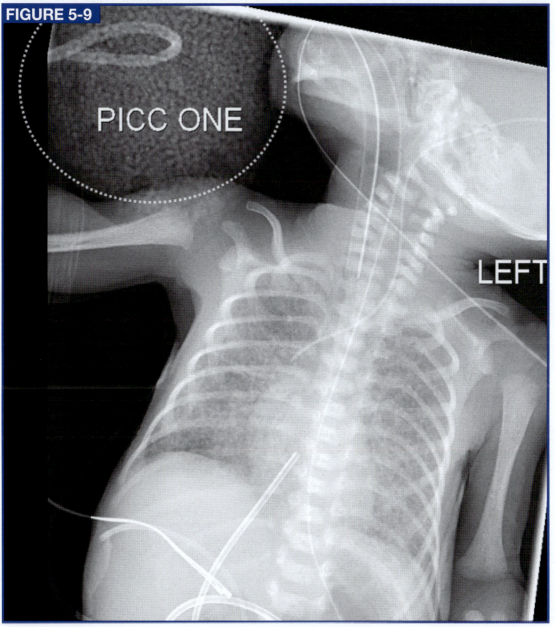

FIGURE 5-9

A plush toy appears as a rounded density with multiple radiopaque dots (dashed circle) in the right upper corner of this image obtained during PICC placement.

OTHER EXTERNAL ARTIFACTS

Tracheostomy Collar

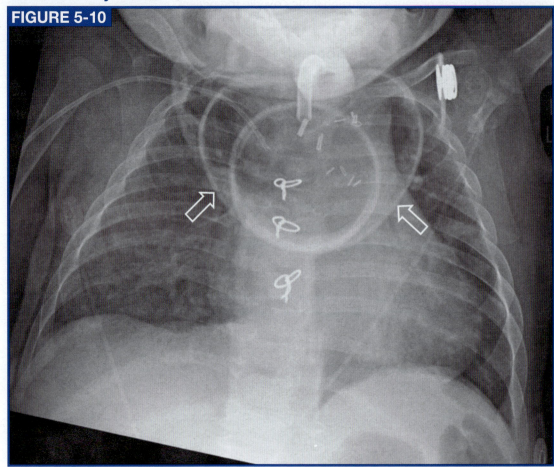

FIGURE 5-10

The superimposed round artifacts centered inferior to the tracheostomy tube (open arrows) represent a tracheostomy collar in this patient with congenital heart disease and chronic respiratory failure.

Umbilical Clip

FIGURE 5-11

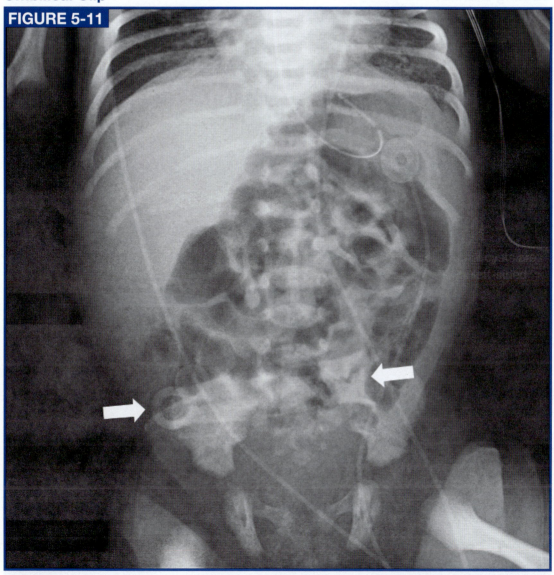

An umbilical clip (arrows) can be seen overlying the lower abdomen of this newborn infant.

Cooling Blanket

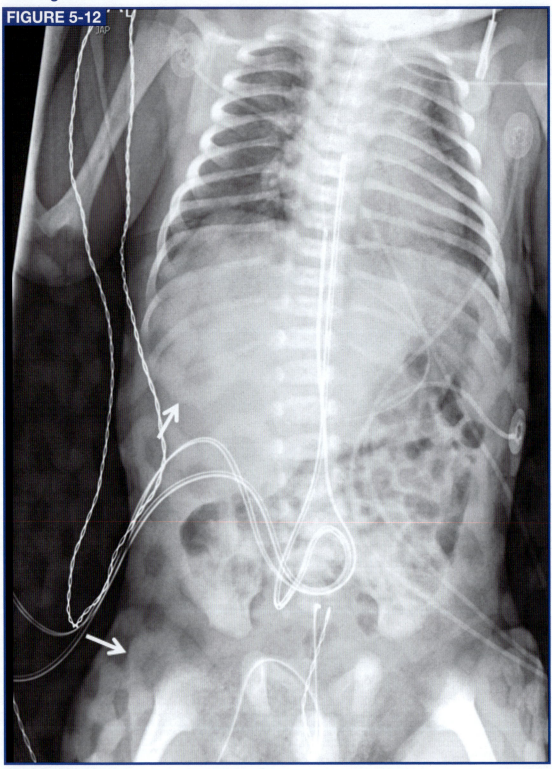

FIGURE 5-12

This overlying waffle-type artifact (arrow) of a cooling blanket, used for patients with hypoxic ischemic injury, is clearly outside the patient, but could obscure subtle findings of the study.

Chapter 6 Case Challenges

CASE 1

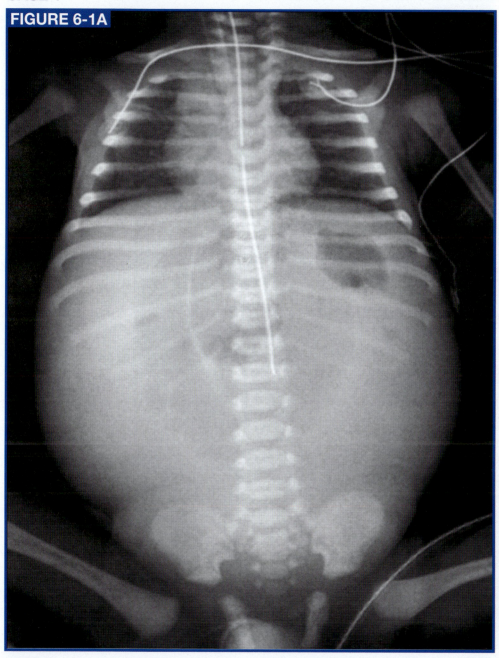

FIGURE 6-1A

History

Preterm neonate with a tense, distended abdomen.

Challenge

Identify the abnormality. What is the next appropriate step?

CASE 1 (continued)

History

Preterm neonate with a tense, distended abdomen.

Challenge

Identify the abnormality. What is the next appropriate step?

Answer

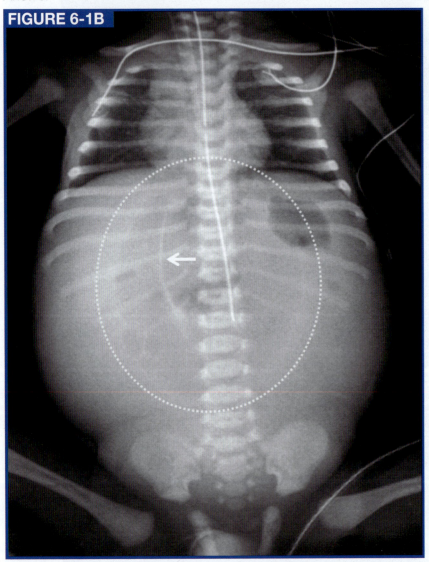

FIGURE 6-1B

The infant has pneumoperitoneum. A large round lucency overlies the central upper abdomen (dashed circle). The falciform ligament is visualized (arrow), which is compatible with a positive "football sign." These findings should prompt immediate surgical consultation.

CASE 2

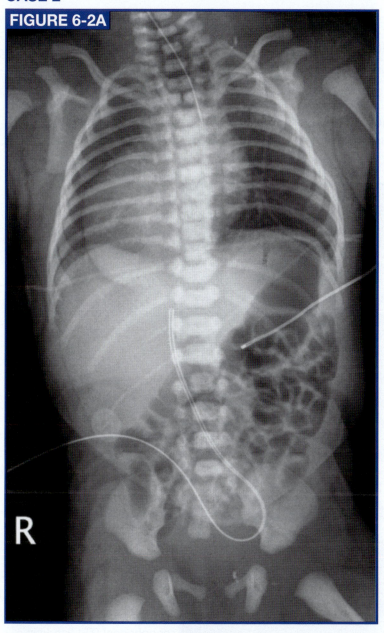

FIGURE 6-2A

History

Newborn who has difficulty feeding. The enteric tube did not easily advance into the stomach.

Challenge

Provide an explanation for the abnormal position of the enteric tube. What other abnormalities are present? Can you name the associated syndrome?

CASE 2 (continued)

History

Newborn who has difficulty feeding. The enteric tube did not easily advance into the stomach.

Challenge

Provide an explanation for the abnormal position of the enteric tube. What other abnormalities are present? Can you name the associated syndrome?

Answer

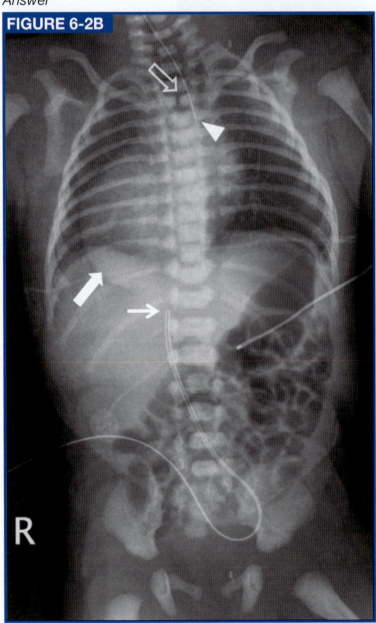

FIGURE 6-2B

In this radiograph of a patient with esophageal atresia, the tip of the enteric tube (arrowhead) projects over a dilated, gas-filled proximal esophageal pouch. The presence of gas-filled bowel loops in the abdomen indicate that a tracheo-esophageal (TE) fistula is present. Vertebral segmental anomalies (open arrow) and dextrocardia (thick arrow) are also present. The patient should be fully evaluated for VACTERL syndrome. Note that the umbilical venous catheter (UVC) is positioned abnormally low (thin arrow).

CASE 3

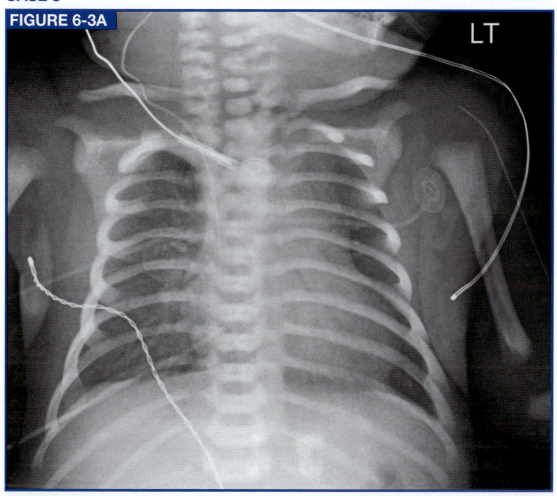

FIGURE 6-3A

History
Newborn infant status post-placement of support lines.

Challenge
Identify which lines have been placed and which are overlying the patient's skin.

CASE 3 (continued)

History

Newborn infant status post-placement of support lines.

Challenge

Identify which lines have been placed and which are overlying the patient's skin.

Answer

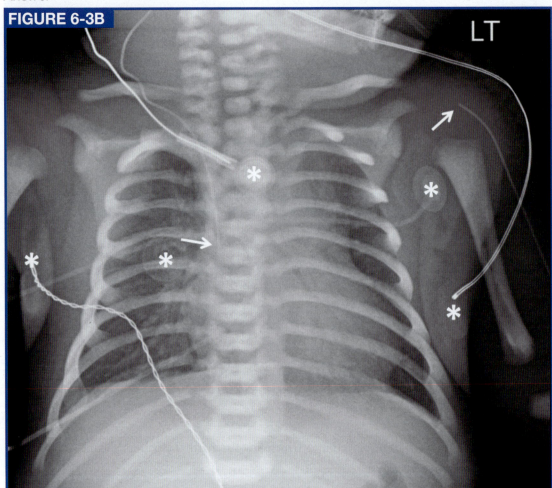

FIGURE 6-3B

Two peripherally inserted central catheters (PICCs) course within the vasculature (arrows). These were placed in the right scalp and the left upper extremity. The remaining radiopaque linear objects, which are thicker, are monitoring leads on the patient's skin (asterisks). Note that the left upper-extremity PICC projects over the soft tissues of the left shoulder. It will need to be repositioned if central location is desired.

CASE 4

FIGURE 6-4A

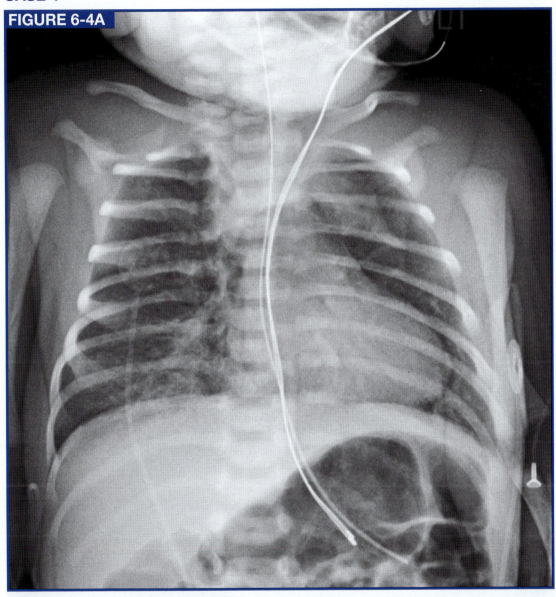

History

Preterm infant with respiratory distress.

Challenge

What accounts for the abnormality in the mediastinum?

CASE 4 (continued)

History

Preterm infant with respiratory distress.

Challenge

What accounts for the abnormality in the mediastinum?

Answer

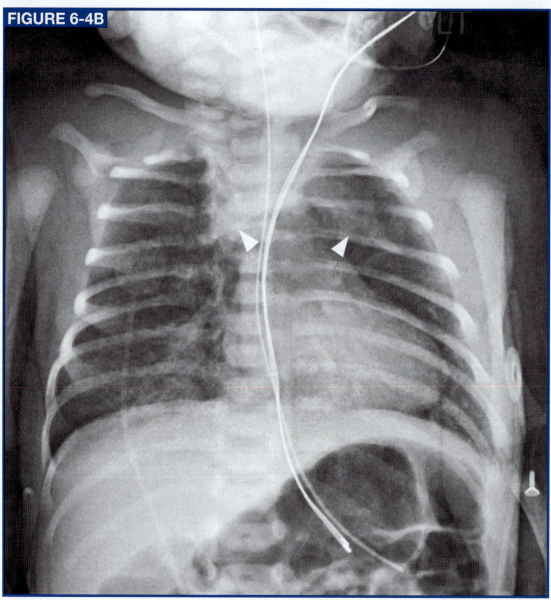

FIGURE 6-4B

The infant has pneumomediastinum. There is abnormal lucency surrounding the heart, particularly superiorly, with associated elevation of the thymic tissue (arrowheads). This appearance of the thymus is characteristic of the "spinnaker-sail sign."

CASE 5

FIGURE 6-5A

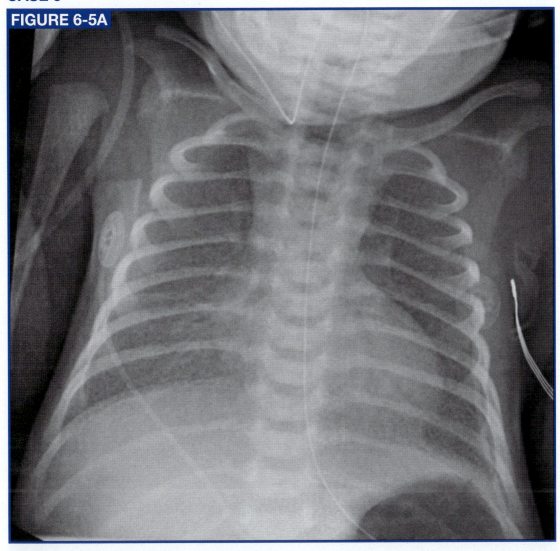

History

Preterm infant born at 29 weeks gestational age with respiratory distress.

Challenge

What lung abnormality is present?

CASE 5 (continued)

History

Preterm infant born at 29 weeks gestational age with respiratory distress.

Challenge

What lung abnormality is present?

Answer

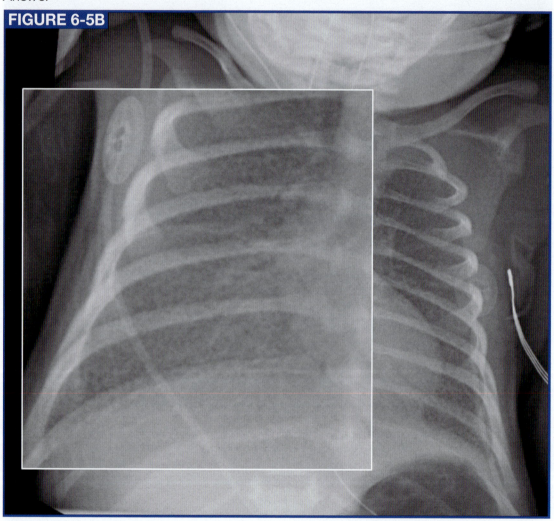

FIGURE 6-5B

Diffuse, granular interstitial densities are present, indicating surfactant deficiency. The heart is normal in size and there are no pleural effusions, making heart failure and pulmonary edema less likely.

CASE 6

FIGURE 6-6A

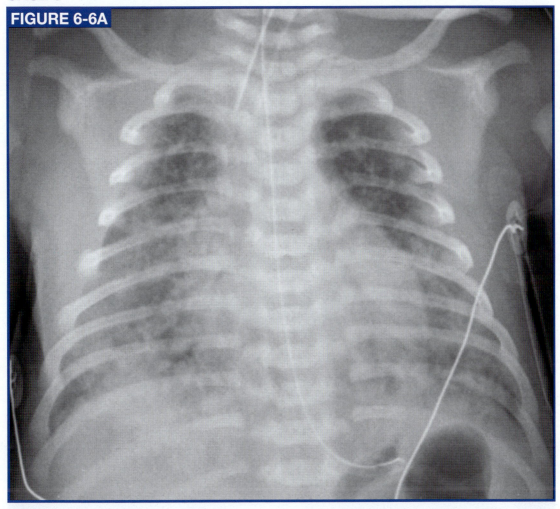

History

Term infant with respiratory failure after birth.

Challenge

There was evidence of fetal distress immediately before delivery. What do the lung findings likely represent?

CASE 6 (continued)

History

Term infant with respiratory failure after birth.

Challenge

There was evidence of fetal distress immediately before delivery. What do the lung findings likely represent?

Answer

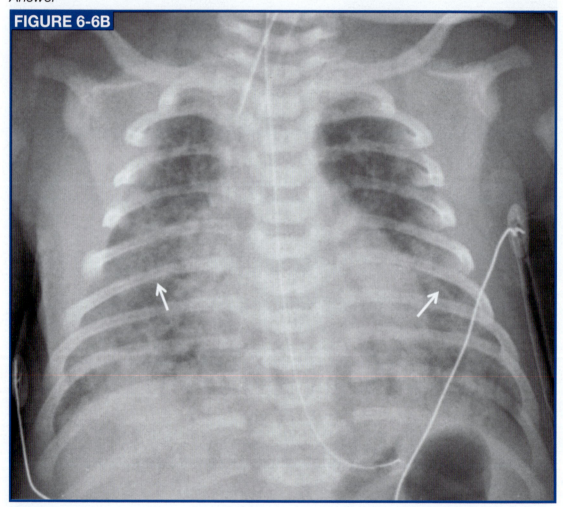

FIGURE 6-6B

Diffuse, coarse (or ropey) interstitial densities are seen throughout the lungs (arrows), with patchy densities seen predominantly at the lung bases. More than six anterior ribs project over the lungs bilaterally, indicating pulmonary hyperinflation. Given the lung findings and the infant's history of fetal distress, meconium aspiration syndrome is likely. The presence of meconium-stained amniotic fluid at delivery would support the diagnosis.

CASE 7

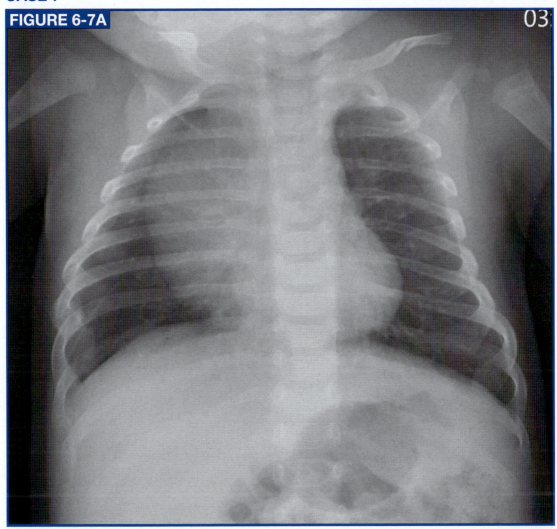

FIGURE 6-7A

History

Term infant with apnea.

Challenge

Describe the abnormality.

CASE 7 (continued)

History

Term infant with apnea.

Challenge

Describe the abnormality.

Answer

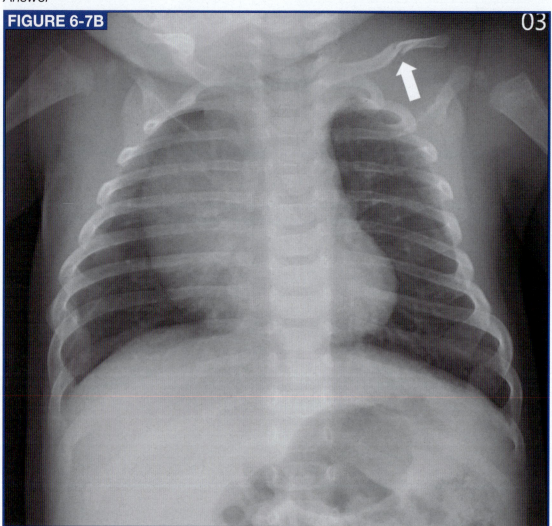

FIGURE 6-7B

Careful inspection of all included osseous and soft tissues is required on all radiographic images. In this case, the salient finding is found on the periphery of the image, an area that can be easily overlooked. A left clavicle fracture (arrow) is present due to a difficult delivery with shoulder dystocia. Most clavicle fractures will heal without complication. However, early identification can prevent confusion should a palpable abnormality develop in this area during healing or if future concern for non-accidental trauma (child abuse) occurs. The mediastinum and lungs are normal.

CASE 8

FIGURE 6-8A

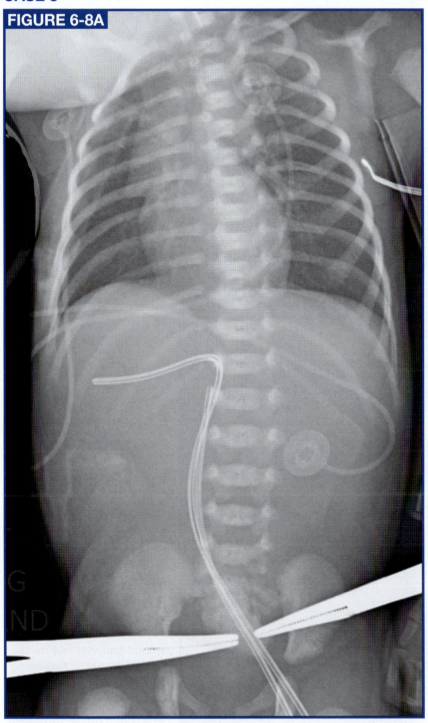

History

Newborn preterm infant with need for parenteral nutrition.

Challenge

Count and describe the position of the UVCs.

CASE 8 (continued)

History

Newborn preterm infant with need for parenteral nutrition.

Challenge

Count and describe the position of the UVCs.

Answer

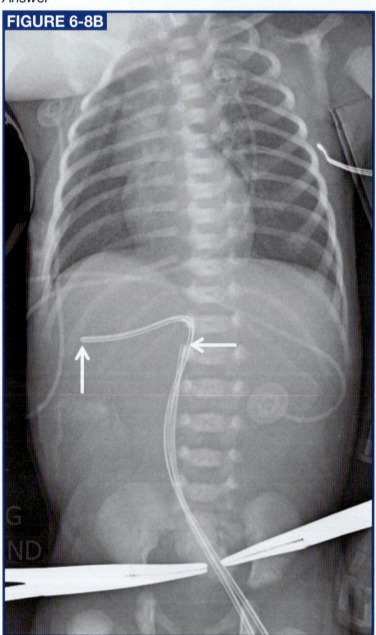

FIGURE 6-8B

Two UVCs have been placed (arrows). One extends into the right branch of the portal vein, with its tip directed laterally toward the right. A second catheter has its tip at the level of L2. Neither catheter is appropriately positioned. Note the hemostat surgical devices overlying the pelvis. The radiograph was obtained in a sterile field.

CASE 9

FIGURE 6-9A

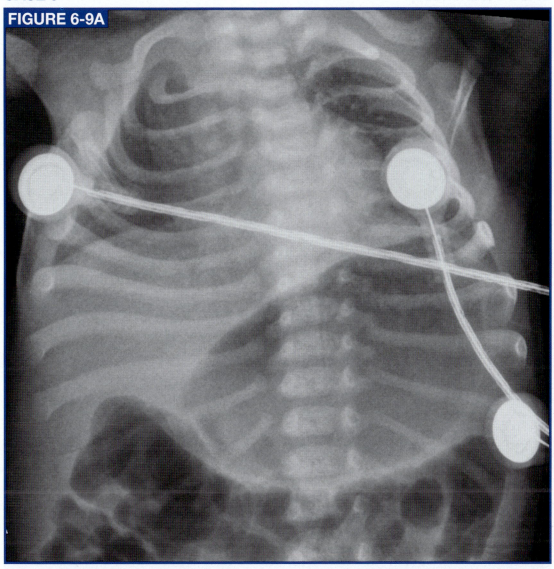

History

Preterm infant with respiratory distress.

Challenge

Explain the cause for the unusual appearance of the ribs.

CASE 9 (continued)

History

Preterm infant with respiratory distress.

Challenge

Explain the cause for the unusual appearance of the ribs.

Answer

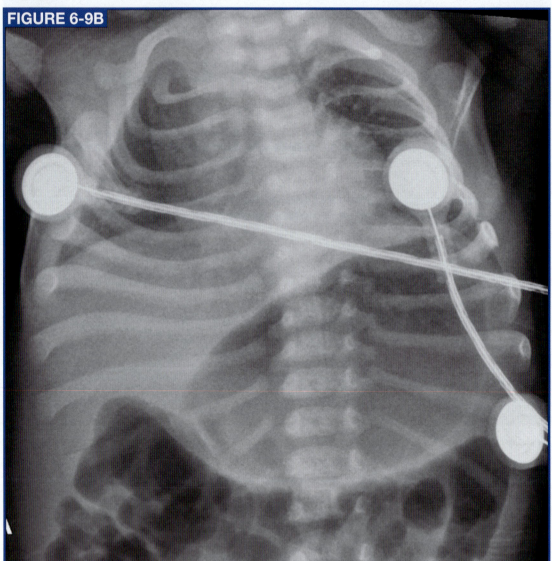

FIGURE 6-9B

The distorted appearance of the ribs is due to the trajectory of the x-ray beam, which is centered on the upper abdomen instead of the chest. The patient is also rotated rightward. The osseous structures would be normal in appearance if the positioning was improved.

CASE 10

FIGURE 6-10A

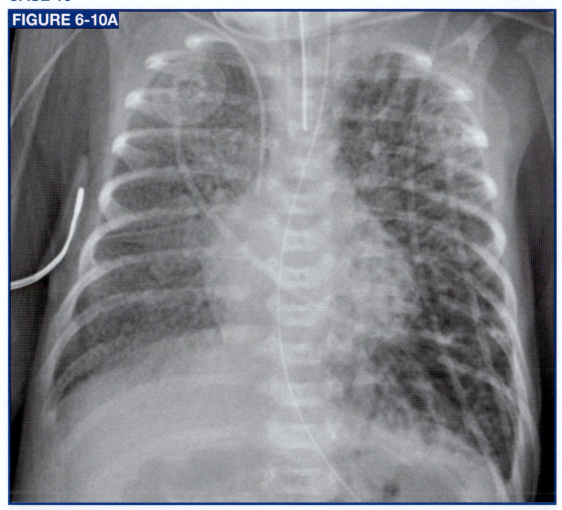

History

Preterm infant with respiratory failure.

Challenge

What lung abnormalities are present? Name one complication that can occur as a result.

CASE 10 (continued)

History

Preterm infant with respiratory failure.

Challenge

What lung abnormalities are present? Name one complication that can occur as a result.

Answer

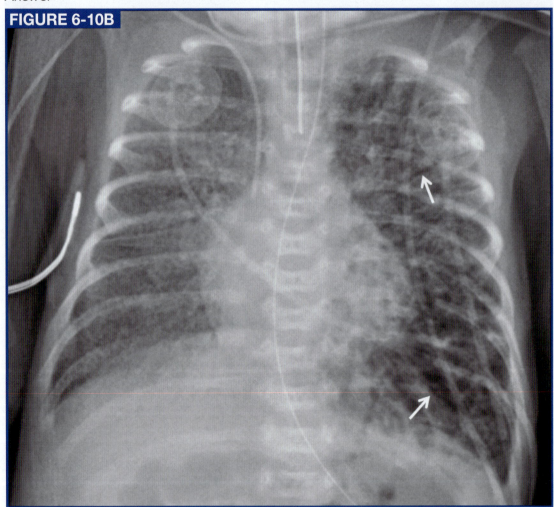

FIGURE 6-10B

The lungs demonstrate diffuse, granular interstitial opacities of surfactant deficiency. There are also asymmetric branching and cystic lucencies throughout the left lung (arrows), compatible with pulmonary interstitial emphysema (PIE). Associated hyperinflation of the left lung is indicative of air trapping. Pneumothorax is one complication of PIE that can occur as air dissects through the interstitium.

CASE 11

FIGURE 6-11A

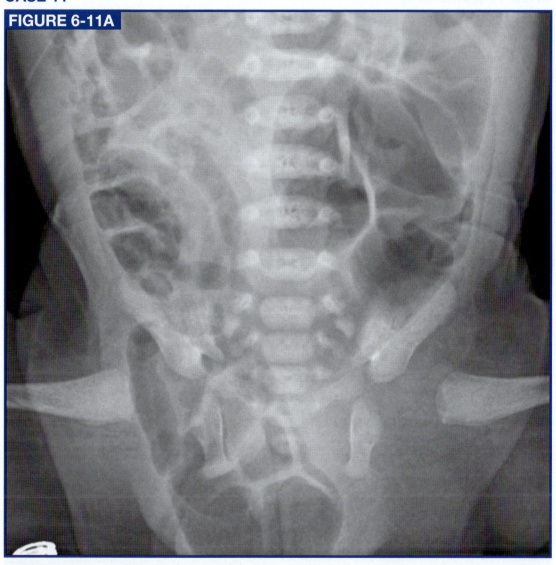

History

Neonate with asymmetric inguinal fold.

Challenge

Identify the abnormality that accounts for physical exam findings of asymmetric inguinal fold.

CASE 11 (continued)

History

Neonate with asymmetric inguinal fold.

Challenge

Identify the abnormality that accounts for physical exam findings of asymmetric inguinal fold.

Answer

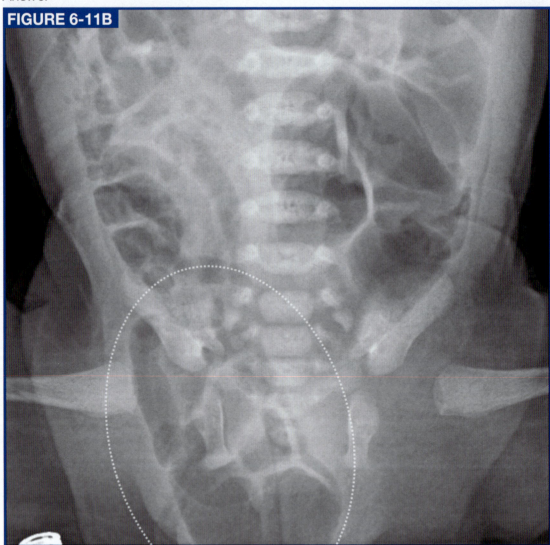

FIGURE 6-11B

The patient has a large, right-sided, bowel-containing inguinal hernia (dashed oval). Inguinal hernias are very common in the premature population. They are often repaired only after all acute illnesses have been resolved, when the patient has grown to a larger size. The bowel can occasionally become incarcerated in the hernia defect, which results in bowel obstruction and requires more urgent attention.

CASE 12

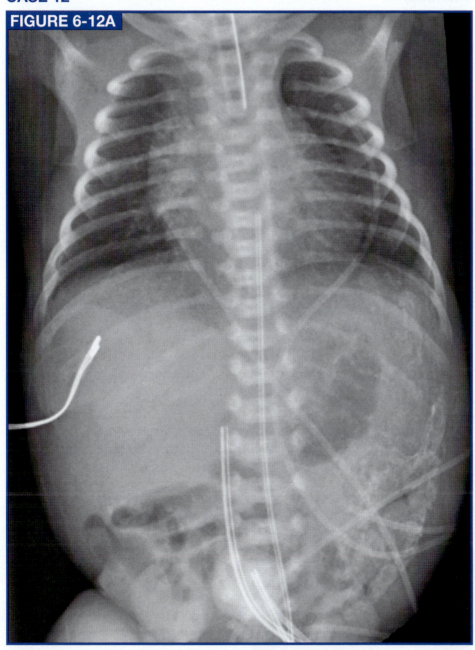

History

Premature infant born at 34 weeks gestational age who has difficulty tolerating feeds.

Challenge

Identify the abnormality in the left abdomen.

CASE 12 (continued)

History

Premature infant born at 34 weeks gestational age who has difficulty tolerating feeds.

Challenge

Identify the abnormality in the left abdomen.

Answer

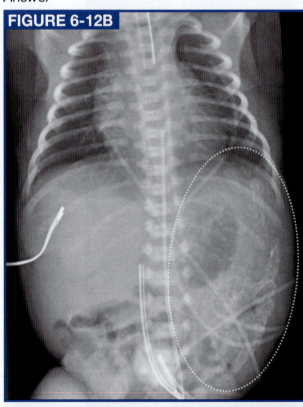

FIGURE 6-12B

There are vague calcifications throughout the left abdomen (dashed circle). Their morphologic appearance and distribution are suggestive of meconium peritonitis from *in utero* bowel perforation. Note the malpositioned UVC, with the tip overlying the inferior liver.

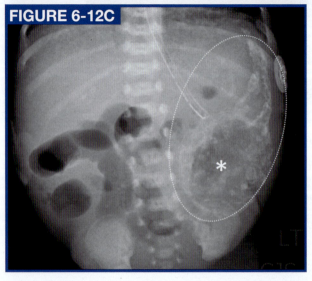

FIGURE 6-12C

A follow-up radiograph obtained approximately two weeks later shows increased density of the calcifications (dashed oval) and an overlying round lucency (asterisk), which are compatible with a contained perforation and meconium pseudocyst formation.

CASE 13

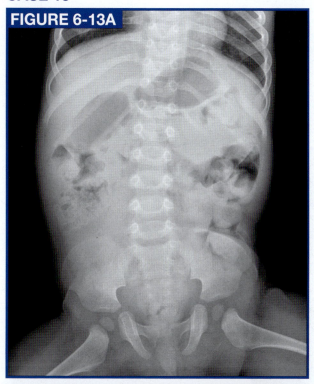

FIGURE 6-13A

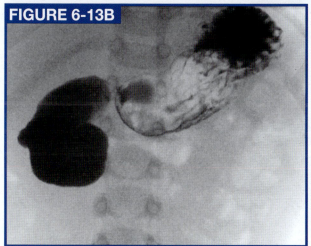

FIGURE 6-13B

History

Patient with chronic emesis and failure to thrive.

Challenge

What is the diagnosis?

CASE 13 (continued)

History

Patient with chronic emesis and failure to thrive.

Challenge

What is the diagnosis?

Answer

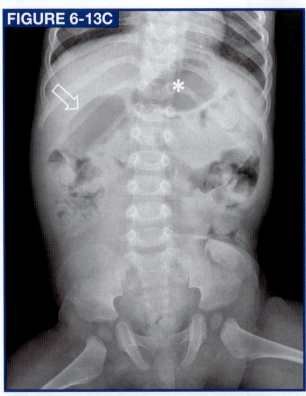

Dilation of the proximal duodenum (open arrow) and a distended stomach (asterisk) are seen on the abdominal radiograph.

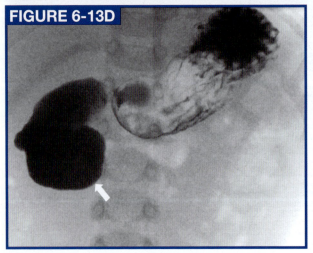

The fluoroscopic upper GI examination reveals a duodenal web (arrow) associated with chronic duodenal obstruction. The stomach is also distended. Although distal bowel gas is present, no contrast passed through the duodenal web during the 20-minute examination due to the severity of the obstruction. Did you notice the ossification of the femoral heads? These images were obtained from a two-year-old adopted child.

CASE 14

FIGURE 6-14A

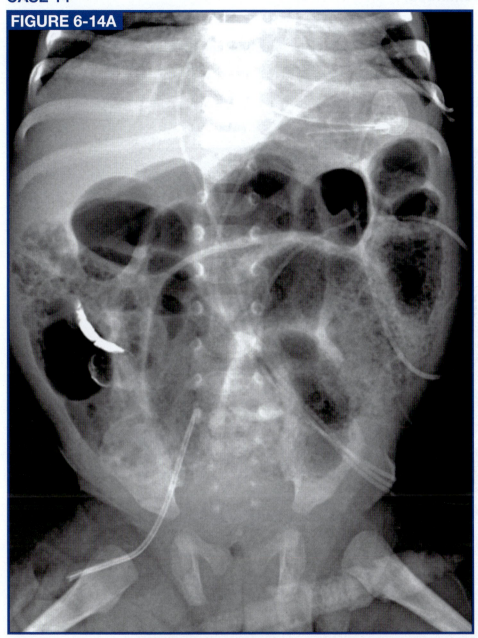

History

Preterm infant with acute onset of abdominal distension and discoloration.

Challenge

What is the diagnosis?

CASE 14 (continued)

History

Preterm infant with acute onset of abdominal distension and discoloration.

Challenge

What is the diagnosis?

Answer

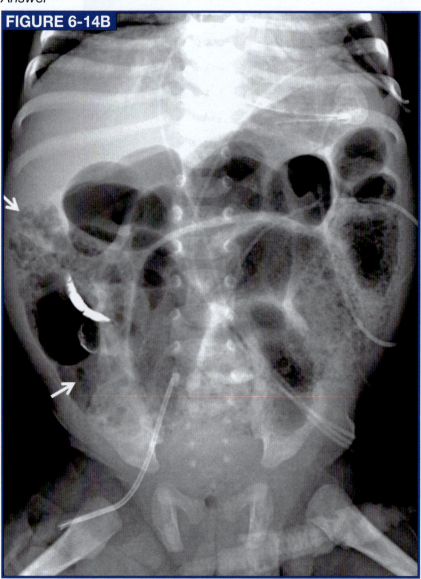

FIGURE 6-14B

The patient has necrotizing enterocolitis. The bowel is diffusely dilated and there are abnormal bubbly lucencies overlying the bowel (arrows), compatible with pneumatosis intestinalis. The patient needs to be followed closely to evaluate for signs of bowel perforation. Note the dense oral contrast material retained in the appendix from a recent upper GI examination.

CASE 15

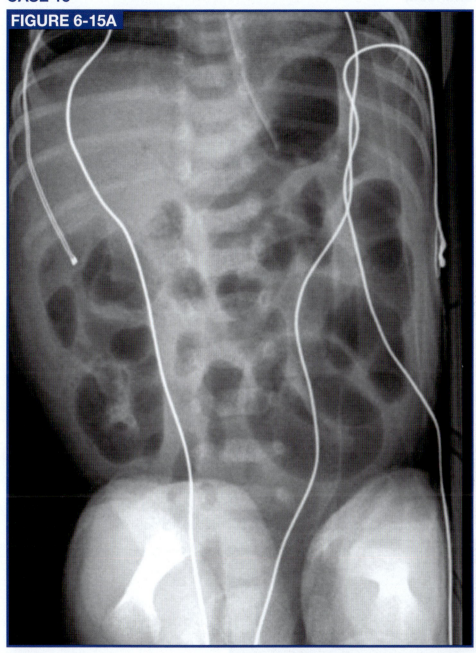

FIGURE 6-15A

History
Preterm infant with bloody stools.

Challenge
What complication of necrotizing enterocolitis is present?

CASE 15 (continued)

History

Preterm infant with bloody stools.

Challenge

What complication of necrotizing enterocolitis is present?

Answer

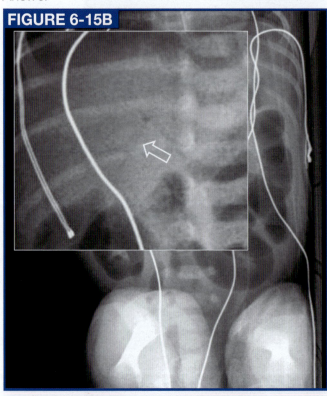

Subtle linear lucencies projecting over the liver indicate portal venous gas (open arrow). If pneumoperitoneum were present, it would likely be seen as a lucency overlying the right lateral margin of the liver on this radiograph, which was obtained in the left-lateral decubitus position.

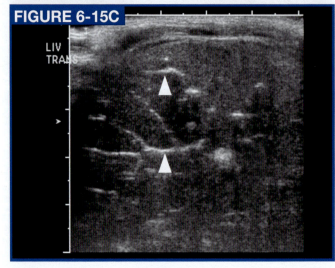

Portal venous gas can also be identified on abdominal ultrasound, and manifests as linear echogenic areas coursing along the portal venous vessels (arrowheads).

CASE 16

FIGURE 6-16A

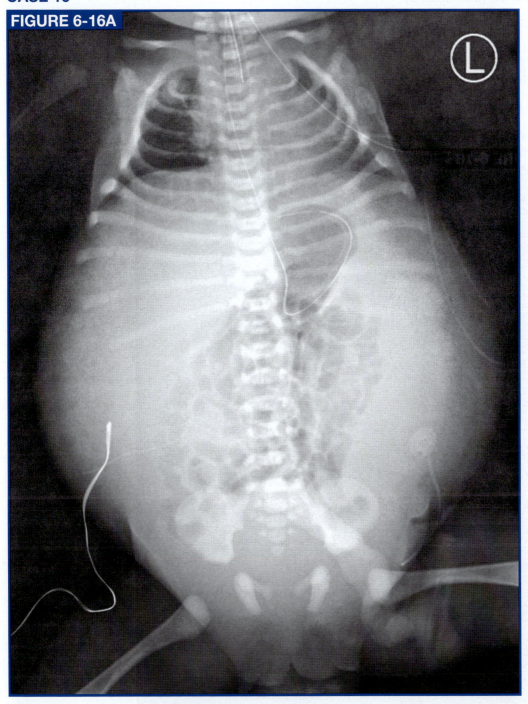

History

Term neonate with respiratory failure.

Challenge

Give two possible explanations why the lungs appear small.

CASE 16 (continued)

History

Term neonate with respiratory failure.

Challenge

Give two possible explanations why the lungs appear small.

Answer

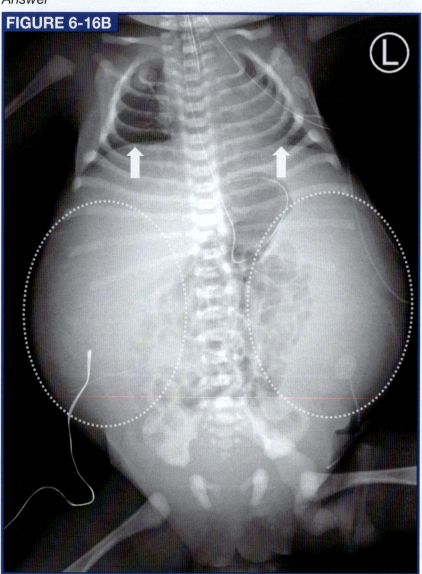

FIGURE 6-16B

This infant has severe bilateral hydronephrosis with enlarged kidneys causing mass effect on the surrounding bowel (dashed ovals). The very small lung capacity (arrows) is due to a combination of factors, including pulmonary hypoplasia related to end-stage renal disease and increased intra-abdominal pressure pushing the diaphragms superiorly. Ascites is also present, which contributes to the centralization of the bowel loops. Note the infant's bulging flanks.

CASE 17

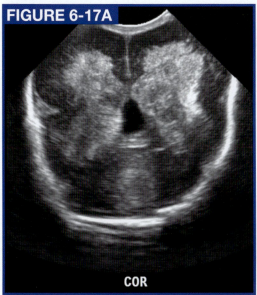
FIGURE 6-17A

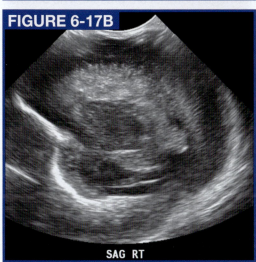
FIGURE 6-17B

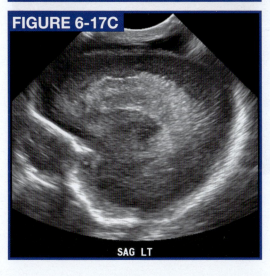
FIGURE 6-17C

History

Preterm infant born at 24 weeks gestational age with metabolic acidosis.

Challenge

Name the diagnosis.

CASE 17 (continued)

History

Preterm infant born at 24 weeks gestational age with metabolic acidosis.

Challenge

Name the diagnosis.

Answer

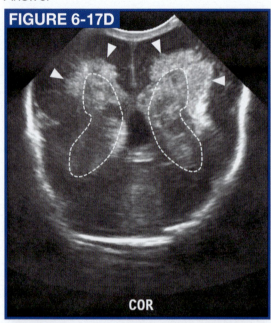

FIGURE 6-17D

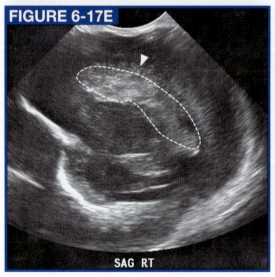

FIGURE 6-17E

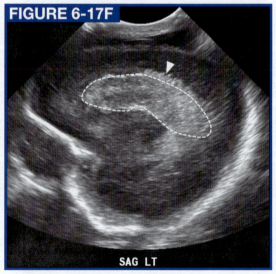

FIGURE 6-17F

Bilateral, grade IV germinal matrix hemorrhages (GMHs) are present. The coronal and sagittal views of the brain show echogenic material compatible with blood products filling the lateral ventricles (dashed outline). Periventricular hyperechoic areas (arrowheads) represent parenchymal hemorrhage. The brain parenchyma demonstrates a very smooth surface, in keeping with history of prematurity. This baby is at risk for post-hemorrhagic hydrocephalus due to the severity of the bleed.

CASE 18

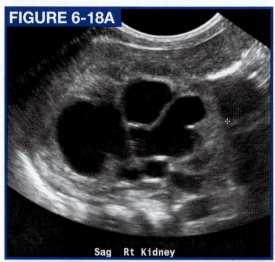

FIGURE 6-18A — Sag Rt Kidney

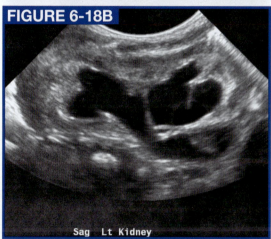

FIGURE 6-18B — Sag Lt Kidney

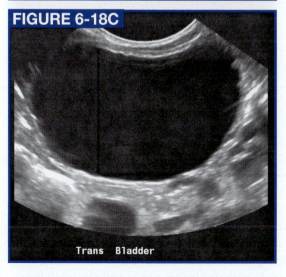

FIGURE 6-18C — Trans Bladder

History

Male neonate with prenatal diagnosis of hydronephrosis.

Challenge

What diagnostic study should be performed next to further evaluate the abnormalities on renal ultrasound?

CASE 18 (continued)

History

Male neonate with prenatal diagnosis of hydronephrosis.

Challenge

What diagnostic study should be performed next to further evaluate the abnormalities on renal ultrasound?

Answer

Voiding cystourethrography (VCUG) should be performed to further evaluate the urinary tract.

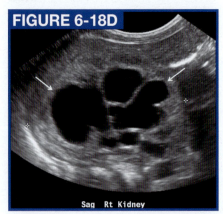

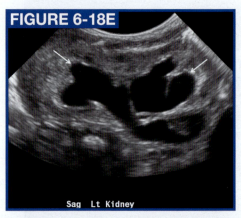

There is bilateral, SFU grade 4 hydronephrosis with severe dilation of the calyces (arrows), as well as parenchymal thinning of the kidneys.

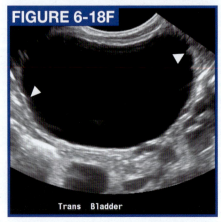

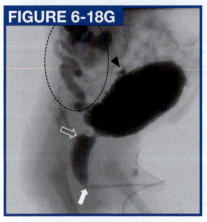

Mild irregularity of the bladder wall is demonstrated (arrowheads), which indicates muscular hypertrophy from chronic bladder outlet obstruction. VCUG will be helpful to further elucidate the cause of the urinary tract dilation, and in a male patient, posterior urethral valves must be ruled out.

Subsequent VCUG shows marked dilation of the posterior urethra, with narrowing at the site of the posterior urethral valves (arrow). The bladder is trabeculated (arrowhead), and there is associated high-grade vesicoureteral reflux. Note that the urinary catheter (open arrow) has retracted into the capacious posterior urethra with voiding.

CASE 19 – CHALLENGE CASE

FIGURE 6-19A

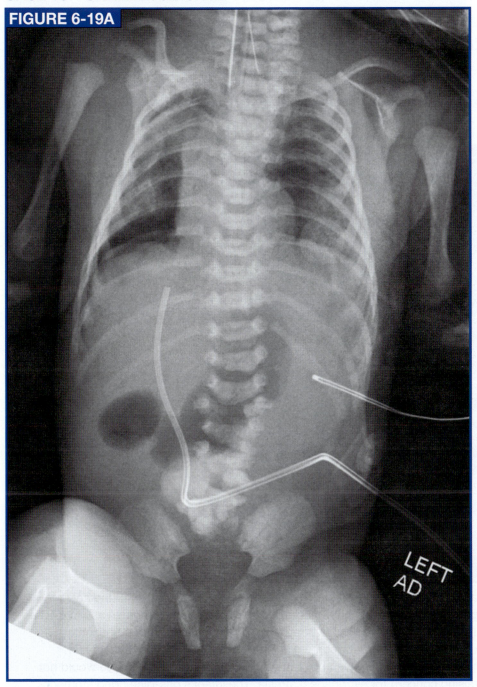

History

Newborn with respiratory distress and abnormal prenatal imaging.

Challenge

Name the abnormalities. What other imaging is emergently required?

CASE 19 – CHALLENGE CASE (continued)

History

Newborn with respiratory distress and abnormal prenatal imaging.

Challenge

Name the abnormalities. What other imaging is emergently required?

Answer

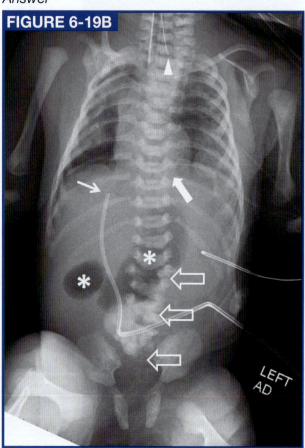

FIGURE 6-19B

The patient has numerous abnormalities. There is increased lucency around the heart bilaterally, suggestive of bilateral pneumothoraces and potential pneumomediastinum. The cardiac silhouette is normal in size but is boot-shaped (thick arrow), with a horizontally oriented apex that raises concern for congenital heart disease (Tetralogy of Fallot, in particular). An enteric tube terminates above the thoracic inlet (arrowhead) and would not pass further, raising concern for esophageal atresia. The infant's gas-distended stomach and dilated duodenum (asterisks) without distal bowel gas are consistent with a complete duodenal obstruction due to duodenal atresia. There are osseous abnormalities (open arrows), including vertebral segmental anomalies and complete absence of the sacrum. In addition, a UVC is malpositioned with the tip overlying the liver (thin arrow), and physical examination reveals no anus. Given the respiratory distress and pneumothoraces, findings raise concern for pulmonary hypoplasia and Potter's syndrome.

Ultrasound of the kidneys should be performed emergently.

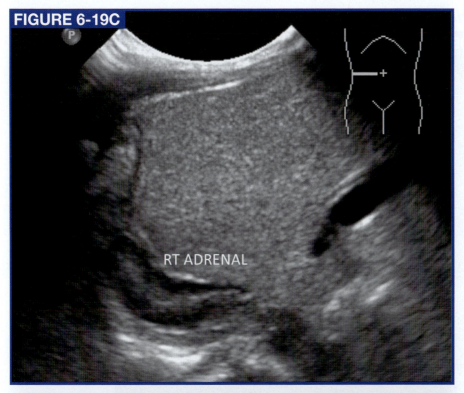

FIGURE 6-19C

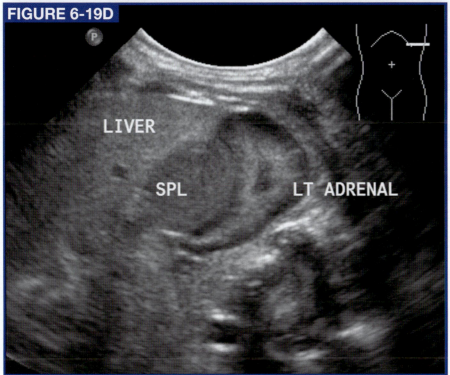

FIGURE 6-19D

Transverse ultrasound images of the right and left flanks demonstrate absent kidneys, with elongated adrenal glands filling the expected location of the kidneys.

CASE 19 – *CHALLENGE CASE* (continued)

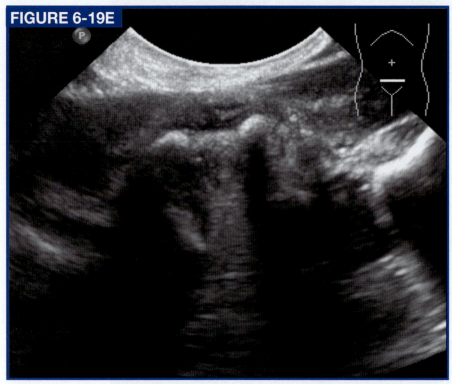

FIGURE 6-19E

An image of the pelvis reveals no fluid in the urinary bladder. The patient has renal agenesis.

The combination of **v**ertebral anomalies, **a**norectal malformation, **c**ardiac defect, **t**racheo-**e**sophageal fistula, **r**enal anomalies, and **l**imb abnormalities is known as VACTERL syndrome.

Given the patient's numerous anomalies and apparent pulmonary hypoplasia secondary to Potter's syndrome and renal agenesis, support was withdrawn.

CASE 20 – CHALLENGE CASE

FIGURE 6-20A

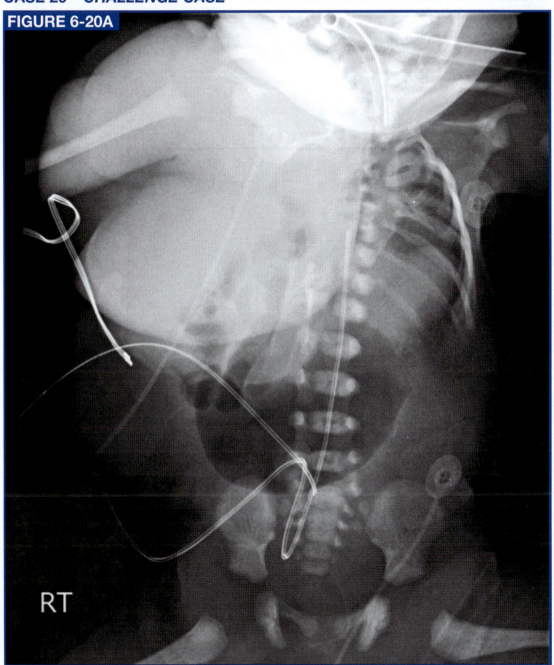

History

Newborn term infant with difficulty ventilating.

Challenge

Name the abnormalities.

CASE 20 – *CHALLENGE CASE* (continued)

History

Newborn term infant with difficulty ventilating.

Challenge

Name the abnormalities.

Answer

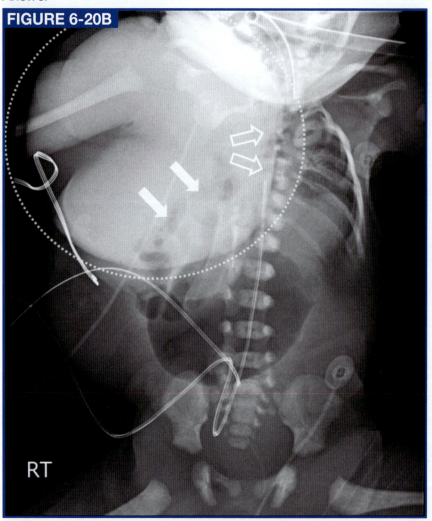

FIGURE 6-20B

This is a very complex case. There is a large soft-tissue density overlying the right upper chest and axilla (dashed circle), which represents a large upper-thoracic myelomeningocele identified by prenatal imaging. There are multiple vertebral segment anomalies in the upper thoracic spine, with associated rib deformities (open arrows). Several right-sided ribs are absent. There is also severe hypoplasia of the right lung tissue. The diaphragm and chest wall are underdeveloped, leading to superior migration of the intra-abdominal structures. Some bowel loops project over the expected location of the lower chest (arrows). The pulmonary hypoplasia and lack of bony support for respiration in the chest wall account for the difficulty ventilating the patient.

Appendix

GLOSSARY OF ACRONYMS

ALARA As low as reasonably achievable
ARPKD Autosomal recessive polycystic kidney disease
BPD Bronchopulmonary dsyplasia
CDH Congenital diaphragmatic hernia
CHD Congenital heart disease
CLO Congenital lobar overinflation
CPAM Congenital pulmonary airway malformation
CT Computed tomography
ECMO Extracorporeal membrane oxygenation
ELBW Extremely low birth weight
ETT Endotracheal tube
GMH Germinal matrix hemorrhage
HPS Hypertrophic pyloric stenosis
IVH Intraventricular hemorrhage
MCDK Multicystic dysplastic kidney
MRI Magnetic resonance imaging
PICC Peripherally inserted central catheter
PIE Pulmonary interstitial emphysema
PPV Positive-pressure ventilation
PVL Periventricular leukomalacia
RDS Respiratory distress syndrome
SFU Society of Fetal Urology
TE Tracheo-esophageal
TORCH syndrome Toxoplasmosis (T), other e.g., syphilis, varicella (O), rubella (R), cytomegalovirus (C) herpes simplex (H)
UAC Umbilical artery catheter
UGI Upper gastrointestinal
UPJ Ureteropelvic junction
UVC Umbilical venous catheter
VACTERL syndrome A disorder that affects multiple systems: vertebral defects (V), anal atresia (A), cardiac defects (C) tracheo-esophageal (TE) fistula, renal anomalies (R), and limb abnormalities (L)
VCUG Voiding cystourethrography
VLBW Very low birth weight

Appendix

GLOSSARY OF ACRONYMS

Suggested Resources

Densen P. Challenges and opportunities facing medical education. *Trans Am Clin Climatol Assoc.* 2011;122:48-58.

Donnelly LF. *Fundamentals of Pediatric Imaging.* 2nd ed. Philadelphia, PA: Elsevier; 2016.

Fuentealba I, Taylor G. Diagnostic errors with inserted tubes, lines and catheters in children. *Pediatr Radiol.* 2012 Nov;42(11):1305-1315. doi:10.1007/s00247-012-2462-7.

Crotty EJ. Neonatal chest imaging. In: Garcia-Peña P, Guillerman RP, eds. *Pediatric Chest Imaging.* 3rd ed. Heidelberg, Germany: Springer-Verlag Berlin Heidelberg; 2014:173-196.

Griscom NT. History of pediatric radiology in the United States and Canada: images and trends. *RadioGraphics.* 1995;15(6):1399-1422.

Huston C. The impact of emerging technology on nursing care: warp speed ahead. *Online J Issues Nurs.* 2013 May 31;18(2):1.

Maxfield CM, Bartz BH, Shaffer JL. A patterned base-approach to bowel obstruction in the newborn. *Pediatr Radiol.* 2013 Mar;43(3):318-329. doi:10.1007/s00247-012-2573-1.

National Institute of Child Health and Human Development (US). *Neonatal intensive care: a history of excellence: a symposium commemorating Child Health Day.* Bethesda, MD: US Dept. of Health and Human Services, Public Health Service, National Institutes of Health; 1992.

Philip A. The evolution of neonatology. *Pediatr Res.* 2005;58(4):799-815.

Siegel MJ. Head and neck. In: Siegel MJ, ed. *Pediatric Sonography.* 4th ed. Philadelphia, PA: Wolters Kluwer/Lippincott Williams & Wilkins; 2011:118-163.

Siegel MJ. Urinary tract. In: Siegel MJ, ed. *Pediatric Sonography.* 4th ed. Philadelphia, PA: Wolters Kluwer/Lippincott Williams & Wilkins; 2011:384-460.

Soto G, Moënne K. Classic chest radiology findings, pearls and pitfalls. In: Garcia-Peña P, Guillerman RP, eds. *Pediatric Chest Imaging.* 3rd ed. Heidelberg, Germany: Springer-Verlag Berlin Heidelberg; 2014:13-30.

Index

A
Abdominal masses, 158-160
Abnormal situs, 161-164
Adrenal hemorrhage, 220-221
ALARA (as low as reasonably achievable) principle, 1
Anechoic, 5
Annular pancreas, 131
Anorectal malformation, 138-140, 274
Anteroposterior view, 3
Arnold Chiari malformations, 196-199
Artifacts, 223-234
    Clothing and diapers, 229-230
    Comfort items, 231
    Mach effect, 225-226
    Monitoring leads and devices, 227-228
    Other external artifacts, 232-234
    Skin folds, 223-224
Ascites, 150-152, 266
Atelectasis, 50-51
Autosomal recessive polycystic kidney disease (ARPKD), 216-217

B
Bell-shaped chest, 78-79
Bowel obstruction, 124-140
    Distal, 136-140
        Anorectal malformation, 138-140, 274
        Imperforate anus, 138-140
    Proximal, 124-135
        Annular pancreas, 131
        Duodenal atresia, 126-128, 272
        Duodenal stenosis, 126-128
        Duodenal web, 129-130, 260
        Hypertrophic pyloric stenosis (HPS), 124-125
        Jejunal atresia, 134-135
        Malrotation with midgut volvulus, 132-133
Bronchopulmonary dysplasia (BPD), 54-55

C
Choroid plexus cysts, 191
Chylothorax, 83
Clothing and diapers, 229-230
Comfort items, 231
Computed tomography (CT) imaging, 5
Congenital diaphragmatic hernia (CDH), 65-69
Congenital heart disease (CHD), 61-64, 272
Congenital lobar overinflation (CLO), 76-77
Congenital malformations, 191-199
    Arnold Chiari malformations, 196-199
    Choroid plexus cysts, 191
    Corpus callosum abnormalities, 192-193
    Dandy Walker malformations, 194-195
Congenital pulmonary airway malformation (CPAM), 70-72
Contrast, 5
Corpus callosum abnormalities, 192-193
Cross-table lateral view, 2

D
Dandy Walker malformations, 194-195
Decubitus view, 4
Density, 2
Distal bowel obstruction, 136-140
Doppler, 5
Duodenal atresia, 126-128, 272
Duodenal stenosis, 126-128
Duodenal web, 129-130, 260
Duplicated collecting system, 209-210

E
Echogenicity, 4
Edema, 187-188
Endotracheal tubes (ETTs), 21-24
Enteric tubes, 110-112
Esophageal atresia, 80-82, 238, 272
Extra-axial hemorrhage, 178-179
Extracorporeal membrane oxygenation (ECMO) cannulae, 32-34

F
Fluoroscopic imaging, 5

G
Gastroschisis, 153-154
Germinal matrix hemorrhage (GMH), 171-175, 268

H
Hydrocephalus, 180-183, 268
Hydronephrosis, 204-207, 266, 270

Hyperechoic, 4
Hypertrophic pyloric stenosis (HPS), 124-125
Hypoechoic, 4

I

Imperforate anus, 138-140
Intraparenchymal hemorrhage, 176-177
Ionizing radiation, 1
Ischemia, 187-188
Isoechoic, 5

J

Jejunal atresia, 134-135

L

Lenticulostriate vasculopathy, 189-190
Line and tube positioning
    Endotracheal tubes (ETTs), 21-24
    Enteric tubes, 110-112
    Extracorporeal membrane oxygenation
        (ECMO) cannulae, 32-34
    Peripherally inserted central catheters
        (PICCs), 25-31, 107-109
    Umbilical artery catheters (UACs), 100-106
    Umbilical venous catheters (UVCs), 92-99,
        250
Lucency, 2
Lung volumes, 18-20

M

Mach effect, 225-226
Magnetic resonance imaging (MRI), 5
Malrotation with midgut volvulus, 132-133
Meconium aspiration syndrome, 60, 246
Meconium peritonitis, 141-143, 258
Monitoring leads and devices, 227-228
Multicystic dysplastic kidney (MCDK), 214-215

N

Necrotizing enterocolitis, 144-149, 262, 264
Neonatal pneumonia, 59
Normal abdominal radiograph, 90-91
Normal chest radiograph, 14-17
Normal head ultrasound, 167-170
Normal kidney ultrasound, 202-203

O

Omphalocele, 155-157

P

Peripherally inserted central catheters (PICCs),
    25-31, 107-109
Periphery, 35-38, 113-118, 248, 276
Periventricular leukomalacia (PVL), 184-186
Pneumomediastinum, 45-47, 242, 272
Pneumoperitoneum, 119-123, 236
Pneumothorax, 39-44, 272
Positioning, 10-13, 88-89
Posterior urethral valves, 211-213, 270
Posteroanterior view, 3
Proximal bowel obstruction, 124-135
Pulmonary hemorrhage, 56
Pulmonary interstitial emphysema (PIE), 48-49,
    254
Pulmonary sequestration, 73-75

R

Radiographic imaging, 2

S

Selection factors of imaging modalities, 6
Skin folds, 223-224
Sonography, 4
Stasis nephropathy, 218-219
Surfactant deficiency, 52-53, 244, 254

T

Technique, 7-9, 87, 165-166, 201-202
Thoracic neoplasm, 84-86
Tracheo-esophageal (TE) fistula, 80-82, 238, 274
Transient tachypnea of the newborn, 57-58

U

Ultrasound imaging, 4
Umbilical artery catheters (UACs), 100-106
Umbilical venous catheters (UVCs), 92-99, 250
Upper gastrointestinal (UGI) imaging, 5
Ureteropelvic junction (UPJ) obstruction, 208

V

Voiding cystourethrogram (VCUG), 6

X

X-ray, 2